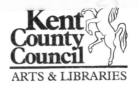

Standards of Care in Anaesthesia

# Standards of Care in Anaesthesia

# Standards of Care in Anaesthesia

**T. H. Taylor** MB BS, FFARCS
*Consultant Anaesthetist, The Royal London Hospital, London;
Member of Council, Medical Protection Society*

and

**D. R. Goldhill** MA, MB BS, FFARCS
*Senior Lecturer and Honorary Consultant, Academic Department of
Anaesthetics, The Royal London Hospital, London*

Foreword by
**Professor Stanley Feldman** BSc, MB BS, FFARCS
*Charing Cross and Westminster Medical School*

Commentary by
**Simon Taylor** MA, MB BChir, Barrister-at-Law
*Pump Court, Temple, London*

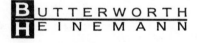

Butterworth-Heinemann Ltd
Linacre House, Jordan Hill, Oxford OX2 8DP

 PART OF REED INTERNATIONAL BOOKS

OXFORD   LONDON   BOSTON
MUNICH   NEW DELHI   SINGAPORE   SYDNEY
TOKYO   TORONTO   WELLINGTON

First published 1992

**British Library Cataloguing in Publication Data**
Taylor, T. H.
    Standards of Care in Anaesthesia
    I. Title II. Goldhill, D. R.
    617.9

ISBN 0 7506 0063 2

**Library of Congress Cataloguing in Publication Data**
Taylor, T. H. (Thomas H.)
    Standards of care in anaesthesia/T. H. Taylor, D. R. Goldhill.
    p.   cm.
    Includes index.
    ISBN 0 7506 0063 2
    1. Anesthesiology – Standards – Great Britain.   I. Goldhill, D. R.
    (David R.)   II. Title.
    [DNLM: 1. Anesthesia – standards.   WD 200 T246s]
    RD80.5.G7T38 1992
    617.9'6'021841–dc20
    DNLM/DLC
    for Library of Congress                                    91–47923
                                                                CIP

Typeset by STM Typesetting Ltd, Amesbury, Wilts.
Printed and bound in Great Britain by Clays Ltd, St Ives, plc

# Contents

# Foreword

## The need for 'standards of care'

It is now thought to be essential that effective medical audit is carried out on all areas of medical practice, and anaesthesia is no exception. In this specialty, as in all others, it is imperative to establish an acceptable minimum standard of care before there can be effective clinical audit. For many leading anaesthetists 'excellence' seems to be the only appropriate goal, but as this standard would be rarely met, audit would, for the majority of practitioners, always reveal only failure. While in no way wishing to advocate anything other than a supreme standard of excellence as a personal and departmental goal in the specialty, it is important that the standard set for purposes of comparison between individuals and departments should be attainable by all the practitioners involved. Thus there will continue to be debate about the possible standards, and this book is a contribution to this debate. It will inevitably produce strong feelings among anaesthetists. Furthermore, in the National Health Service in the United Kingdom, financial constraints currently impinge on all activities. The implicit assumption that all doctors have a duty to perform to the best of their ability in the interest of a particular patient is, in some ways, being supplanted by the need to conform to the standards and practices that the corporate body of anaesthetists perceives to be correct. Fortunately, at the present time other important individuals and organizations, including health service managers, have little influence on clinical practice, except of course, lawyers in cases of negligence. However, the pressures resulting from the corporate bodies of anaesthetists will challenge many previously held convictions, and to avoid confusion it is essential to understand the basic tenets on which these corporate ideas are founded, so the individual can reach his or her own conclusions on the way they will affect their personal practices.

The objective of any practitioner when giving an anaesthetic to a patient is quite unambiguous, even if sometimes difficult to define. It is, of course, to provide safe and sensible treatment before, during and after an operative or invasive procedure. The problem of defining standards begins when there are several possible alternative methods which will achieve this aim.

The past decade has seen an increase in the number of regulatory bodies setting standards of practice, in addition to those set by the judgments delivered by the courts of law in cases of alleged negligence. The regulatory bodies include professional associations, colleges and universities, but there is also a considerable input from the reports of enquiries and working parties, such the Confidential Enquiry into Perioperative Deaths (Buck, Devlin and Lunn, 1987) and that set up by the Royal College of Surgeons of England and the College of Anaesthetists (1990) on postoperative pain. The recommendations of the professional bodies and the reports of working parties tend to assume the status of enacted laws, largely because of the pressures to conform within them to avoid claims of negligence for not so doing. Thus the medico-legal pressure is to perform within the framework of the acceptable majority opinion, which soon becomes the acceptable standard in all circumstances. The limitation of freedom associated with rigid adherence to these standards is further encouraged by the examination system through which each practitioner must pass. In this particular forum it is very easy for the accepted answer to an examiner's question to become equated with correct practice. As a result, and quite inadvertently, alternative anaesthetic regimes and practices may be interpreted as unacceptable by the examinee. Thus influences are developing that are progressively limiting the freedom of the individual to perform as he thinks best in a particular circumstance, and pressure is building to conform with recommended, or in some cases mandatory, regimes, without allowing the individual to evaluate them in his own way.

But these are not the only influences affecting the clinical practitioner. The patient has the same objective as the anaesthetist, that is, a safe and trouble-free anaesthetic and recovery. But, either through the private health insurance companies or the National Health Service administrators, restrictions are placed on the time and cost of treatment. Pressure is exerted for the cheapest and most expedient form of medicine, irrespective of what the doctor wishes, the academic institutions recommend or the lawyers demand. Thus practising anaesthetists are caught on the horns of a dilemma, under pressure to compromise in the way they conduct anaesthesia and therefore to ignore in part their prime responsibility to treat each patient to the best of their ability and in a manner they think appropriate, irrespective of time and money.

It would seem that there are two options for future development in this dilemma. The first, and perhaps the easier option to follow, is the acceptance of and blind obedience to increasingly intrusive mandatory treatment regimes. This will progressively strip doctors of the freedom to make decisions based on medical knowledge, anaesthetic training and technical skills. By enacting a series of anaesthetic responses to all conceivable (or inconceivable) eventualities, the authoritative body will reduce the doctor to the level of a mere technician, responding to situation A with treatment B and so on. Critical incidents will be monitored as though each were exactly reproducible and its outcome predictable, and a standard management regime will be enforced. If the pulse rate falls to 50 beats per minute, atropine is given. If more than eight extrasystoles a minute occur, lignocaine is given intravenously, or perhaps propanolol. If ventilation down an endotracheal tube becomes difficult, give adrenaline. These are all actual examples of rules presently in force in various anaesthetic departments throughout the world, often with the predictably disastrous results.

The alternative approach is to define the objectives and the limits of proper safe practice and to indicate the line of thought that will produce a minimum acceptable standard of care. In this way the goals are set but the precise method of achieving, or even exceeding, the desired objective is left to the clinician. This method is intellectually more appealing and allows flexibility to adapt treatment to changing circumstances, patient pathology, available facilities and anaesthetic experience. It also admits the heresy that perhaps even the most august body of wise men meeting in conclave do not always produce the most sensible treatment regimes. The history of medicine and anaesthesia demonstrates that medical arrogance of this kind has occurred in the past and is always counter-productive. This is well illustrated by the medical fashions that have masqueraded as the 'best' treatment in past years, not least in our own specialty. Indeed, some of the presently accepted shibboleths in anaesthetic practice have little scientific basis, and will eventually be discarded. The number of hours of simple fluid restriction imposed on a patient before an elective anaesthetic is perhaps a good example.

This book sets out to include all the relevant material with sufficient references to enable the anaesthetist to perceive what is a poor standard of care for his or her patients, with the material arranged in a logical sequence. It will enable the reader to eschew dogma and to recognize that there are differing ways for an anaesthetist to achieve the desirable end of a safe operation and recovery. It also shows that mandated regimes may be irrelevant, for what may be safe in one set of circumstances may be unsafe in another. The future direction of anaesthetic practice will depend on which path is followed by the profession as a whole. By indicating the requirements for the care of a patient by the anaesthetist this book contributes to a debate that will influence the very nature of the future practice of the specialty.

# References

Buck, N., Devlin, H. B. and Lunn, J. N. (1987) *Report of the Confidential Enquiry into Perioperative Deaths*, Nuffield Provincial Hospitals Trust/King's Fund, London
Royal College of Surgeons of England and College of Anaesthetists (1990) *Report of the Working Party on Pain after Surgery*, RCS, London

*Stanley Feldman*

# Preface

Now, *here*, you see, it takes all the running *you* can do, to keep in the same place. If you want to get somewhere else, you must run at least twice as fast as that!

Lewis Carroll, *Through the Looking-glass*

The number of textbooks of anaesthesia available in the English language is large and ever growing. Before augmenting the total, authors and publishers must have a valid reason for doing so. The idea for this volume originated with Stanley Feldman, and is based on a concern we all shared. We felt that too many rules and regulations relating to patient care and safety were being enunciated by the various official bodies and these were reinforced by the examination system through which all trainees must pass. Although the adoption of these rules and regulations is not mandatory, on occasion too little effort is expended on verifying the assertions made. The present authors are certain that, given the correct information, the modern generation of anaesthetists are quite able to plan and administer safe anaesthetics to the wide range of patients that come under their care. This should be done by evaluating the relevant literature and adapting current practice accordingly, thus minimizing the need for compulsion or rule books, but building on the scientific training that anaesthetists now receive. In this book we have tried to review those matters relating to the care of a patient in the perioperative period that is properly the province of the anaesthetist. The information needed is set out in such a way that an informed choice can be made, with sufficient references appended for additional reading if further knowledge is sought. We hope this will lead to the adoption of the proper technique of anaesthesia for each patient, and contribute to patient safety. The final chapter, by Simon Taylor, is a commentary on the material in the factual chapters. It is hoped this will put the medico-legal aspects of care into perspective.

*T. H. T.*
*D. R, G.*

# 1

# Preoperative assessment I: General principles

## The decision to operate

### Responsibility of the initiator

The initiator of an anaesthetic may be a surgeon, a physician, an obstetrician, a radiologist or one of the many other specialists that call upon anaesthetic services. When a clinical decision is made which will lead to a patient's being given an anaesthetic, then that patient will be exposed, albeit rarely, to a risk of complications, some serious or permanent, or even death. The risk depends on the operation, investigation or procedure to be undertaken, but is also affected by the physical status of the patient. Thus the initiator of the process, as well as the anaesthetist administering the anaesthetic, should be aware of the risk and the factors that contribute to it. Any advice given to the patient should consider the benefit of the procedure compared to the attendant risk, recognize alternative treatment that may exist, and consider how, where and when the intervention should proceed to ensure maximum safety.

The decision to perform surgery is influenced by factors other than the patient's illness or condition. These include available resources, whether the patient is privately insured, the social class of the patient, the practice of the surgeon or referring physician, and the patient's expectations. Experience from the United States has shown that where procedures are carried out on a fee-for-service basis excessive surgery may be performed (Bates, 1990); and of course special considerations should apply when performing operations that are essentially 'cosmetic' and do not directly result in physical benefit to the patient.

### Responsibility of operator and anaesthetist

The doctors caring for the patient must have the appropriate skills, knowledge and experience to perform the procedure to be undertaken.

This means that adequate supervision and advice must be available to doctors in training, while senior staff must know their own limitations. With the increasing specialization of surgery and anaesthesia it is no longer possible for one person to be expert in all areas of practice. The Confidential Enquiry into Perioperative Deaths (CEPOD) (Buck, Devlin and Lunn, 1987) found unnecessary deaths occurred because some surgeons operated for conditions for which they were not trained or which were beyond their field of primary expertise. One of the major recommendations of this report was that operations should only be performed by consultants or junior surgeons who have had adequate training in the specialty relevant to the operation. The same considerations must apply to the doctor administering the anaesthetic.

Patients have the right to assume that they will be looked after by competent and caring doctors. In the United Kingdom, patients admitted under the National Health Service commonly have the impression that the consultant under whom they have been admitted will perform the operation, although this is clearly not the case, does not always happen, and indeed could not always happen under the present British state system. The consultant does, however, have the responsibility of ensuring that the operation is carried out by someone who is competent to do so, and this is done by appropriate delegation to a more junior doctor.

## Available facilities

Safe surgery and anaesthesia should only be planned if adequate facilities and support staff are available. The facilities required will depend on the procedure to be undertaken but will also be dictated by the potential problems that a particular patient may present. For example, the requirements for open heart surgery will obviously be different from those needed to perform dental extractions in healthy patients. The complexity of surgery and anaesthesia, and the importance of proper equipment, supplies, monitoring and trained staff, dictate that only in exceptional circumstances will an anaesthetic be given outside properly equipped areas of a hospital or day centre. In a modern hospital, a fully staffed and equipped anaesthetic room, resuscitation room, operating room and recovery area should be available at all times for genuine emergency surgery. The facilities should be complemented by a high dependency area or intensive care unit.

## Timing

Surgery, both elective and emergency, should be performed as far as possible during normal working hours. The CEPOD report highlighted the increased risk to patients who had surgery outside of this period (Buck, Devlin and Lunn, 1987). During the working day support services such as radiology and pathology are available and all the facilities of the hospital should be properly staffed. If elective work continues after scheduled operating times then the resources may not be available to run the emergency services. It is the responsibility of the hospital administration to reduce such over-runs to a minimum.

Emergency surgery carries a higher patient mortality than similar elective procedures. The patients for emergency surgery are, in general, sicker and less well prepared than those for elective surgery. Additionally, in the National Health Service this more demanding work is often left to surgical and anaesthetic trainees without immediate consultant supervision. Ideally, as the CEPOD report recommends, emergency surgery should be performed during working hours and by experienced surgeons with experienced anaesthetists.

Seasonal factors influence the medical condition of some patients. Chronic bronchitis and hay fever are two examples which readily come to mind. Wherever possible, operative procedures and anaesthesia should be scheduled for a time when the patient could be expected to be least affected by these conditions. There are certain changes to lifestyle or habits that may benefit the patient referred for surgery and it is also important to optimize control of medical conditions, some of which can affect outcome from surgery and anaesthesia. These are discussed in Chapter 3. If the patient needs several operations, investigations or treatments in the immediate future, then the significance of each should be considered and the patient's management planned so as to treat the most serious pathologies first and to avoid duplication of investigations and consultations.

Patients have a commitment to their normal employment, holidays to arrange and a duty to their families. All these should be considered when deciding on a date for an elective operation. One advantage of day care surgery for appropriate procedures is that appointments can be made some time in advance and can, in general, be kept. Admission does not depend on bed availability and the timing of the procedure will not be affected by the unpredictable nature of major and emergency surgery.

## Transplant surgery

The transplant surgeon must only be involved in planning surgery once donor organs are available. The decision to perform tests of brain stem function must not be influenced, or even be thought to be influenced, by the potential for organ donation. Members of the transplant team must therefore never be involved in the diagnosis of brain stem death in a potential organ donor nor should they be involved in decisions about the timing of the harvest of organs from donors who have not yet been declared 'brain dead' by others. A conflict of interest can occur when an anaesthetist is involved in the care of a potential donor in the intensive care unit and is then likely to anaesthetize the recipient in the operating theatre, or when a surgeon counsels live donors and also looks after the patient who is to be the recipient.

## Surgical and anaesthetic risk

An appreciation of the factors contributing to perioperative mortality and major morbidity is necessary if problems are to be identified and appropriate decisions taken when planning an operative procedure for a patient.

### Surgical risk

Surgical mortality is largely related to the operation to be undertaken but is increased when the procedure is prolonged, during emergency operations, in the aged and when the physical status of the patient is poor. In addition to these unavoidable factors, the CEPOD report highlighted other circumstances that contributed to preventable mortality related to surgery. Surgery was the sole cause in 7% of the deaths, and about 20% of these were due to inappropriate operations, poor preoperative management or the wrong grade of surgeon operating, and were considered to be preventable (Buck, Devlin and Lunn, 1987).

### Anaesthetic risk

It has been estimated that anaesthesia alone is responsible for about one death in 10 000 operations, and perhaps 80% of these deaths are preventable. Factors thought to influence these deaths include failure of judgement by the anaesthetist, failure of the anaesthetist in knowledge or application of that knowledge, lack of care and skills, failure to check equipment or inadequate equipment, and lack of supervision or facilities. More specifically, they include omitting prophylaxis for pulmonary thromboembolism in patients at risk (although this is also a surgical responsibility), inadequate monitoring, inappropriate doses of drugs, and failure of a trainee to consult a senior colleague (Buck, Devlin and Lunn, 1987). Further discussion of anaesthetic-related morbidity and mortality is to be found in Chapter 8.

# Preoperative assessment

## Benefits of preoperative assessment

### Anticipating problems

When the patient presents for an anaesthetic assessment a decision has already been made that an operation is necessary. The anaesthetist has the responsibility for ensuring that the patient's physical status is appropriate for that operation and that any relevant information from the history, examination or investigations is obtained.

The risks of anaesthesia increase with the presence and severity of co-existing disease. If problems are identified preoperatively then it may be possible to improve the patient's health or alter anaesthetic management so as to reduce mortality and morbidity. The assessment also delineates baseline function against which intraoperative and postoperative changes can be compared.

### Planning action

As a general rule a patient undergoing an operation should be in optimum physical condition within the constraints imposed by any disease process or urgency of operation. The information gained from the preoperative assessment guides preoperative action to achieve this goal and provides an indication of the facilities, skills and assistance required for the procedure. Advice to the patient or further investigations, consultations or treatment are sometimes desirable. It may be wise to delay, alter or cancel the proposed procedure and it is useful to have the opportunity to consider a particular technique, to consult a relevant textbook or article, or to seek advice from a colleague.

### Psychological benefits

A preoperative visit can be used to provide information to the patient on the conduct of the anaesthetic and the potential hazards and side effects. If the visit is undertaken by the anaesthetist who will be giving the anaesthetic then a rapport between patient and doctor may be achieved. A pre-anaesthetic visit has an anxiolytic effect that may be as effective, if not more so, than a premedicant (see Chapter 3). This process also educates the patient and clarifies the role the anaesthetist plays in treatment.

### Safety

If the anaesthetist meets the patient before the operation there is much less risk of mistakes in identity, and also in performing the wrong procedure or operating on the wrong side. Not only are gross errors avoided in this way but if there are undesirable sequelae after the procedure the patient will be less likely to take action against a doctor who has made a preoperative visit and discussed potential problems. It may also be easier for a doctor to defend his actions if there is written evidence in the notes that problems have been anticipated and action taken to manage them.

## Place and time of preoperative assessment

It is important that there is sufficient time between assessment and surgery to be able to organize any further investigations and consultations, and to allow for appropriate therapy to be instituted. If this time is too long the patient's condition may have changed, thus invalidating the assessment. If waiting lists are long and the operation will occur months or years after the decision to proceed, a further full assessment will be required shortly before surgery. As a general rule we suggest that for patients with stable disease no more than one month should elapse from assessment and investigations until surgery. For patients with unstable conditions the assessment will remain valid for a shorter time. Economic influences dictate that patients are admitted to hospital with only a short interval before scheduled operating time and it is essential that adequate arrangements for assessment are made for patients who require considerable preoperative work-up.

### Assessment by surgeon

The surgeon should make a preliminary assessment of potential perioperative problems and initiate investigations if required. The suitability of a patient for anaesthesia and the choice of anaesthetic technique is ultimately the decision of the anaesthetist. This decision will depend not only on the patient's medical condition but will take account of the urgency of the surgery and the requirements of the surgeon. If delays and cancellations are to be avoided the surgeon should recognize potential problems that may affect the anaesthetic and be able to consult with anaesthetic colleagues at an early stage in order that the patient can benefit from the advice given. It is therefore necessary for the surgeon to have some appreciation of the factors that affect the anaesthetic and thus influence postoperative morbidity and mortality.

It may seem desirable for patients to change their life style, but this is often a sacrifice they find difficult to undertake. In these circumstances any benefits from stopping smoking, for example, will have to be set against the frustration of the patient, and turmoil that the patient might inflict on relatives and friends.

## Anaesthetic assessment clinics

In some hospitals anaesthetic departments run a clinic which patients attend shortly before surgery. The advantages are that patients can be given specific times for assessment during the normal working week, arrangements can be made for required investigations to be performed and reported upon, and time can be allowed for further consultations and to make any special arrangements that may be necessary for the patient's stay in hospital. Thus this system recognizes the importance of the anaesthetist and the anaesthetic preparations, and provides time and facilities for a proper assessment.

There are, however, disadvantages in this system and it will not be appropriate for all patients. The anaesthetic assessment clinics are only suitable for procedures where a sufficient interval is available to allow attendance before admission to hospital. Patients undergoing urgent or semi-urgent surgery have an increased perioperative mortality and morbidity and will often present unusual or complex problems. They will not benefit from such a clinic. Clinic attendance means that patients have to make one or more extra visits to hospital. This is inconvenient for patients and expensive for the hospital because of the costs of providing clinic facilities and support staff. It is most unlikely that arrangements can be made so that the assessment is always performed by the anaesthetist who will look after the patient at surgery. Thus if the patient is to be prepared for surgery, any assessment, including choice of investigations and treatment, will have to be acceptable to the doctor who ultimately gives the anaesthetic. The assessment should therefore be performed by an experienced anaesthetist, who might, however, be of more value giving anaesthetics in the operating theatre. For the assessment to be widely accepted a patient may have more investigations than considered necessary by the anaesthetist at the time of operation, thus increasing expense. Finally it is also possible when the patient eventually comes to surgery that the anaesthetist concerned at that time may consider the preparation inadequate and may therefore delay or cancel the procedure. If this happens the benefits the preoperative assessment clinic was supposed to bring will be negated.

If the patient is in good health – for example, American Society of Anesthesiologists (ASA) classification I or II – and the operation does not require any specific preoperative preparation, then the anaesthetic assessment is unlikely to affect the pre-admission management of the patient. Referring these patients to an assessment clinic is of little value and is a waste of resources.

## Screening questionnaires

Questionnaires are a useful and efficient way of screening for potential problems and for answering routine preoperative questions (Pearson and Jago, 1981; Rollason and Hems, 1981). Questionnaires can be filled in by patients, nurses, doctors or non-medical staff. They are also very suitable for computer-aided completion by the patient, and there is some evidence that not only can they be as good at reaching a diagnosis as a doctor, but the patient is more likely to be truthful with the computer about certain facts, such as the amount of alcohol or tobacco consumed. Once completed, the questionnaires can be used as the basis for the medical history. Although they have the advantage of ensuring that specified questions are covered, they are rigid, and may provide misleading information if misunderstood or wrongly completed by the patient. By awarding scores to factors such as age, smoking history, obesity, diabetes or hypertension, it is possible to identify patients to whom special attention should be paid (Playforth *et al.*, 1987).

An example of a screening questionnaire is given in Table 1.1.

Table 1.1   An example of a preoperative screening questionnaire

Patient's Name:                          Age:                          Weight:

1.  Have you had an anaesthetic before?                                    YES/NO

2.  If YES when was it and what was the operation?

3.  Have you or your family had any problems with anaesthetics?       YES/NO
        If YES please specify.

4.  Have you taken any medicines within the last 6 months?            YES/NO
        If YES please specify.

5.  Are you allergic or sensitive to any drugs or food?               YES/NO
        If YES please specify.

6.  Have you suffered from any of the following?
        If YES please give details.

| | | | |
|---|---|---|---|
| a. Heart disease | YES/NO | j. Kidney disease | YES/NO |
| b. Shortness of breath | YES/NO | k. Jaundice | YES/NO |
| c. Chest pain on exertion | YES/NO | l. Diabetes | YES/NO |
| d. Rheumatic fever | YES/NO | m. Thrombosis | YES/NO |
| e. High blood pressure | YES/NO | n. Epilepsy | YES/NO |
| f. Chest disease | YES/NO | o. Arthritis | YES/NO |
| g. Bronchitis | YES/NO | p. Easy bruising | YES/NO |
| h. Asthma | YES/NO | q. Any other severe illness | YES/NO |
| i. Tuberculosis | YES/NO | | |

7.  Have you false teeth, caps, crowns, or bridge?                    YES/NO
        If YES please specify

8.  Do you smoke?
        If YES please give details                                    YES/NO

9.  Do you drink alcohol regularly?                                     YES/NO
     If YES please give details

10.  Have you suffered any recent illness from which you do not feel fully recovered?
     (coughs, colds, flu, etc.).                                        YES/NO
     If YES please give details

---

## Assessment on the ward

The majority of patients admitted to the hospital for elective and emergency surgery are seen and assessed after admission to a surgical ward. If the need for extra preoperative preparation has been foreseen, or the operation is of some magnitude, they may be admitted a day or two before the operation. In most cases, however, the patients are admitted the day before surgery or, because of the need to save inpatient costs, increasingly on the day of the operation.

In poorly organized units it is not unknown for an anaesthetist to go to see a patient for the first time on the evening before an operation only to discover there are major anaesthetic risk factors which have not been reported despite the patient's having been on the ward for several days or sometimes even weeks. All too often in these cases specialist advice has been sought from other doctors. It is sometimes forgotten that an expert opinion on preparation for an anaesthetic can only be obtained from an anaesthetist. Thus if a patient for surgery presents potential problems an anaesthetic opinion should be sought as soon as the patient is admitted. It is then for the anaesthetist to decide whether additional medical opinion should be obtained.

With the working day of an anaesthetist as presently organized in the United Kingdom, it is often not possible to undertake preoperative ward rounds until after the previous day's operating has finished. Visits in the late afternoon or evening are inconvenient and are sometimes too late to arrange further tests or consultations. To overcome this the house surgeon is usually expected to initiate the necessary investigations, identify potential problems and communicate with the anaesthetist concerned. It is important that they appreciate the preoperative considerations of interest to the anaesthetist. House surgeons show a poor understanding of some anaesthetic-related aspects of care (Carnie and Johnson, 1985), and no anaesthetist should assume that the preoperative assessment by the house surgeon has addressed all relevant points. When the ward assessment is finally completed there should be a clear note of the findings, also indicating the investigations that have been arranged, and when the results will be available.

Ideally the doctor administering the anaesthetic should see patients preoperatively, and work schedules should be designed to allow for this. If admissions are on the same day as surgery this may be difficult without the understanding and cooperation of colleagues. When this ideal arrangement is not possible, a routine and effective method must exist for ensuring an adequate pre-anaesthetic assessment is performed and for informing the patient's anaesthetist of any important problems that emerge.

For all patients, a relevant history should be taken, an examination performed and the important findings, including details of the investigations ordered, briefly summarized in the notes. The records should include the time and date of the assessment and a legible signature of whoever carried it out. These details must be accessible and easily interpreted, and the anaesthetist if he so wishes should be able to question the doctor who performed the assessment.

### Assessment for emergency surgery

Preoperative assessment must not be neglected for patients about to undergo emergency surgery. The risks of emergency surgery are greater than for elective procedures. In addition, it may be necessary to resuscitate the patient before induction of anaesthesia, making the time for preparation of the patient longer than usual. The anaesthetist should be involved at an early stage in the management of the patient, and have a say in the final decision on the best time to start the operation.

The extent of the assessment will depend on the time available, as in the sick patient resuscitation takes priority over history and examination. Usually there will be time to take a short, relevant history, perform a brief examination, and arrange for the essential investigations, even if the results of these will not be available before induction of anaesthesia.

### Assessment in the anaesthetic room

It is always desirable for the anaesthetist to see the patient before arrival in the operating theatre and every effort should be made to organize admissions and operating lists to allow this. Furthermore, the patient should have been given information about the conduct of the anaesthetic and have had an opportunity to ask questions about the procedure. The time and opportunity to perform preoperative assessments in this way are sometimes not available for 'same day' admissions, day care surgery, emergency surgery or when additions or changes are made to the operating list. When an emergency procedure is to be performed the urgency may be such that the first opportunity to assess the patient will be in the operating theatre. Nevertheless, we believe that ideally an assessment by the anaesthetist should be performed before the patient comes to theatre, and to leave this important function until the anaesthetic room is to depart from a proper standard of care.

*Assessment for day care surgery*

An increasing number of patients are subjected to surgery on a day care basis. If selected minor procedures are performed on young patients in excellent health, then assessment of patients can safely take place on the day care unit shortly before surgery (Cooper, 1989).

However, day care surgery need not be confined to this select group of patients. ASA III and even ASA IV patients may also be suitable, and with appropriate management it has been estimated that some 50% of all elective surgery can be performed in this way. For this percentage to be achieved, some of these patients will require assessment before the day of operation, and this needs to be considered when arranging a time for surgery. To maximize day care facilities, all suitable patients should be carefully selected, with a firm rejection of those who are not suitable. The initial assessment can be by telephone, questionnaire or from the general practitioner, but in those patients with potential problems preoperative attendance at an anaesthetic assessment clinic will be necessary.

## Staff performing the preoperative assessment

The person who performs the anaesthetic assessment is not always the anaesthetist who is to give the anaesthetic for the operation. If the patient is admitted to the ward prior to the day of surgery, a house surgeon will perform the initial assessment when completing the admission notes. In an anaesthetic assessment clinic it may be an anaesthetist or nurse. In a day care setting questionnaires may be used. It is also customary for nursing staff to complete an admission chart for their own use, and this often duplicates medical notes.

The essential elements of the preoperative assessment are the relevant history, an appropriate examination and the ordering of indicated investigations, the results of which must be recorded when received. It is important that the assessment is relevant both to the surgery and the anaesthetic.

Ideally the anaesthetic assessment should be performed by the doctor who will administer the anaesthetic. These advantages are detailed under the benefits of the preoperative assessment. If the assessment is carried out by another doctor the anaesthetist administering the anaesthetic should whenever possible see the patient before operation and check or complete the assessment. He should be satisfied that the appropriate preoperative preparation has been made, including the administration of preoperative medication and treatment.

# References

Bates, T. (1990) Avoiding inappropriate surgery: discussion paper. *Journal of the Royal Society of Medicine*, **83**, 176–178

12    Standards of Care in Anaesthesia

Buck, N., Devlin, H. B., Lunn, J. N. (1987) *Report of the Confidential Enquiry into Perioperative Deaths*, Nuffield Provincial Hospitals Trust/King's Fund, London

Carnie, J. and Johnson, R. A. (1984) Clinical anaesthetic knowledge amongst surgical house staff. *Anaesthesia*, **40**, 1114–1117

Cooper, G. M. (1989) Day-case surgery. *Current Opinions in Anaesthesiology*, **2**, 713–716

Pearson, R. M. G. and Jago, J. H. (1981) An evaluation of a pre-operative anaesthetic assessment questionnaire. *Anaesthesia*, **36**, 1132–1136

Playforth, M. J., Smith, G. M. R., Evans, M. and Pollock, A. V. (1987) Pre-operative assessment of fitness score. *British Journal of Surgery*, **74**, 890–892

Rollason, W. N. and Hems, G. (1981) Preoperative assessment for outpatient anaesthesia. *Annals of the Royal College of Surgeons of England*, **63**, 45–49

# 2

# Preoperative assessment II: History, examination and investigations

## Anaesthetic history and examination

The patient's history and clinical examination are the most important elements of the preoperative assessment, and of these, the history is likely to provide the anaesthetist with the most useful information. If the history is carefully taken and examination performed properly, laboratory investigations will reveal little that has not already been suspected or detected. To take a history and perform an examination is safe, cheap and effective, but the detail of the assessment will depend on the health of the patient and the nature of the surgery contemplated. The patient's response to an anaesthetic is determined primarily by the presence and severity of co-existing medical disease. It is not within the scope of this book to list all the effects that medical conditions may have on the conduct of an anaesthetic; moreover, this information can be found in general textbooks. However, some selected conditions are discussed later in this chapter as an illustration of the relevant history and examination that should be obtained as well as a demonstration of the interreactions with anaesthesia that will, in some cases, entail increased risk to the patient.

The person conducting the assessment must be aware of the anaesthetic implications of medical conditions. For example, practical difficulties may be likely at intubation when rheumatoid arthritis affects a patient's mandible or neck, or with obtaining an accurate indirect measurement of blood pressure from the arm of a morbidly obese subject. The uptake, distribution, metabolism and excretion of anaesthetic agents may be altered by lung, renal or hepatic disease. Anaesthesia in turn affects certain organs. The cardiovascular system is obviously an example where agents have varying effects on myocardial function and perfusion. Anaesthetics will also influence the nervous system by altering intracranial pressure or, as with enflurane or methohexitone, by being epileptogenic. Therefore it is the duty of the anaesthetist when performing a preoperative assessment to discover the important factors that will interreact with an anaesthetic. In addition to the patient's medical history the necessary information also includes the patient's attitude and mental state, drug history, known allergies and information on hereditary diseases, as well as the relevant examination and investigations.

## *History*

One of the best ways of obtaining a relevant anaesthetic history is with a series of questions. A list of possible questions is shown in Table 2.1. If there are positive responses to some of these questions then further details may have to be elicited by direct questioning. In this way one question may lead to another.

Table 2.1    Questions to elucidate history which may affect anaesthesia

A.   **Previous and current history**
   1.   Are you in generally good health?
   2.   Are you active for your age?
   3.   Have you any heart or breathing problems?
   4.   Do you get short of breath?
   5.   Do you get any chest pain?
   6.   Do you have high blood pressure?
   7.   Have you ever had a heart attack or rheumatic fever?
   8.   Do you suffer from faints, or epilepsy?
   9.   Have you ever had jaundice or liver problems?
   10.  Do you have, or have you had, any other medical problem that we have not discussed?
   11.  Have you any false teeth, loose teeth, or capped teeth?
   12.  When did you last drink or eat?

B.   **Family history**
   13.  Are there any illnesses in your family that can be inherited?
   14.  Has anyone related to you had any problems with anaesthetics?

C.   **Anaesthetic history**
   15.  Have you had any previous anaesthetics?

D.   **Drug history**
   16.  Do you smoke?
   17.  Do you drink alcohol?
   18.  Do you take any medication of any sort?

E.   **History of allergy**
   19.  Do you have any allergies?

The doctor taking the history should observe the patient while the history is taken as this can often give important clues to further relevant questions. For example, nicotine-stained fingers will be a reminder to ask about the smoking history, and visible arthritis should lead to an examination of the patient's ability to open the mouth and to flex and extend the neck. It is important to consider the underlying pathological condition, for a patient with bowel cancer, for example, may be anaemic, malnourished and deficient in fluid and electrolytes and the history and examination should be directed to cover these points. The drug history is important as it identifies current medical conditions. The specific indication for each drug needs to be ascertained because some drugs have a dual use, for example a diuretic may be given for hypertension or cardiac failure, and beta blockers for control of blood pressure and angina.

## Previous and current history

The anaesthetist must discover relevant past or present illnesses as there are many conditions which are associated with increased perioperative mortality or morbidity. These include previous illnesses which may leave permanent damage, such as rheumatic fever or tuberculosis, as well as problems that are current at the time of the anaesthetic. The history may influence the choice of anaesthetic technique or agents, and action may be necessary in the preoperative period to correct or improve the patient's condition. The most obvious illnesses that profoundly affect outcome from surgery and anaesthesia include a recent myocardial infarction, congestive cardiac failure, severe angina, disorders of cardiac rhythm and renal dysfunction. Other determinants of outcome from surgery and anaesthesia include old age and the need to perform emergency surgery. These considerations are discussed more fully later in the chapter.

In addition to the illnesses that have an impact on the conduct of an anaesthetic, the patient may also have specific anxieties. For example, many patients, especially children, wish to avoid injections, and others may fear a mask induction or have a terror of being aware and paralysed during a general anaesthetic. Lastly as part of the review of the current history the anaesthetist should record a dental history.

## Family history

The family history may reveal information of importance to the anaesthetist, as inherited conditions, including some that have little impact on the patient during normal activity, may require appropriate action to be taken when anaesthesia is contemplated. Conditions that may be revealed by the history include malignant hyperthermia (Ellis, 1990), cholinesterase abnormalities, porphyria, dystrophica myotonica and abnormalities of haemoglobin including sickle cell disease and thalassaemia. If there is a family history of these illnesses enquiry must be made for details of problems previously encountered by other members of the family. The problems associated with malignant hyperthermia and haemoglobinopathies are considered later in the chapter. Cholinesterase abnormalities are not associated with any pathology but may considerably prolong the action of the depolarizing muscle relaxant suxamethonium which is broken down by plasma cholinesterase. Certain types of porphyria contraindicate the use of barbiturates, and several neuromuscular disorders including dystrophica myotonica are associated with complications from the use of muscle relaxants.

*Patient's anaesthetic history*

If the patient has previously undergone an anaesthetic it is vital that information is sought on the administration and outcome from the anaesthetic. The patient may have particular fears and preferences based on previous experience and will also be able to indicate if there were any perioperative problems such as postoperative nausea and vomiting, headache, sore throat, or the complication of a deep vein thrombosis (DVT). This information will assist in planning the present anaesthetic in order to anticipate problems and avoid complications, and by giving an explanation one can allay the fears of the patient. If the patient's notes are available from previous procedures the anaesthetic record must be examined. This will document the techniques and anaesthetic agents previously used and it may explain or expand on problems that the patient has already mentioned. Any problems during the anaesthetic or in the immediate postoperative period should have been clearly stated on the anaesthetic chart, as should have routine information on airway management and use of anaesthetic agents. Such information will include the size of endotracheal tube, if inserted, the degree of difficulty of airway control and intubation, and the use of inhalational anaesthetic agents, and of these it is particularly important to note whether halothane was administered. If there was a serious adverse reaction to a drug given during an anaesthetic it should be clearly described in the record of this anaesthetic. Patients should obviously be aware whether they suffered any life-threatening reaction such as malignant hyperthermia or severe anaphylaxis, but even in these cases there can be confusion about the precise sequence of events. A prolonged neuromuscular block after suxamethonium caused by abnormal cholinesterase should not endanger a patient's life, and may not even affect the course of a long anaesthetic, so it is always useful to ascertain if suxamethonium was administered and was followed by normal spontaneous recovery of muscle power. When referring to the history of previous anaesthetics, if nothing else it is always reassuring to discover that the process was uneventful.

If the patient has undergone a general anaesthetic within the previous 3 months this should lead to caution in the choice of volatile agent, and a repeat administration of halothane is to be avoided. Unexplained postoperative jaundice after any anaesthetic must lead to enquiry as to the possible role of halothane. Elevated postoperative temperature may also indicate liver damage and, because it is rarely possible to be certain of the cause of the pyrexia, once again repeat halothane is best avoided. Because halothane has been widely used until recently, if no previous anaesthetic records are available, it is wise to assume that halothane was given. As other agents are available, the risk of 'halothane hepatitis' can be avoided by not using the drug (Blogg, 1986). The use of halothane for repeat anaesthetics in children probably does not carry danger of the same magnitude as does administration in adults. There are few reports of halothane hepatitis in the very young and several surveys support the use of this agent (Wark, 1983; Brown, 1985). Although halothane may be considered by some to have advantages over other volatile agents for anaesthesia in children, the risks involved should still be considered when an inhalational anaesthetic is planned (Kenna et al., 1987).

## Drug history

Any drugs the patient takes may affect the conduct of an anaesthetic and it is essential that the anaesthetist should be fully aware of them well before the time of induction. The drug history will also identify active medical conditions for which the patient is receiving treatment. Many drugs interreact with anaesthetic agents, and it may be necessary to discontinue, modify or to maintain drug therapy in the perioperative period, although the route of administration will sometimes need to be altered. Many other substances habitually taken by the patient are in effect drugs, and therefore smoking habits, consumption of alcohol and, if suspected, the abuse of potent nonprescription drugs (Wood and Soni, 1989) should be recorded as they may modify the anaesthetic technique. Table 2.2 lists some of the drugs that have potential anaesthetic interreactions.

## History of allergies

Patients may know they have an 'allergy' to specific foods or drugs and careful enquiry should be made to confirm the nature of the symptoms and signs. Patients are not always aware of the medical

**Table 2.2    Groups of drugs with potential anaesthetic interreactions**

| Drug | Effect |
|---|---|
| *1. Cardiovascular drugs* | |
| Beta-blockers | Cardiovascular instability if stopped prematurely. Potential for bronchospasm |
| Calcium channel blockers | Enhanced negative inotropic and chronotropic effects with some volatile anaesthetics |
| Diuretics | Hypokalaemia provoking arrhythmias and prolonged neuromuscular blockade. Obtain serum $K^+$ in chronic users |
| Digoxin | Increased arrhythmias especially with hypokalaemia |
| *2. Antibiotics* | Aminoglycosides may potentiate neuromuscular block and induce microsomal enzymes |
| *3. Psychopharmacological drugs* | |
| Monoamine oxidase inhibitors | Hypertension especially with pethidine |
| Tricyclic antidepressants | Increased arrhythmias with some volatile anaesthetics. Care with exogenous catecholamines |
| Lithium | Potentiation of neuromuscular block. Toxicity with diuretics and dehydration |
| Antiepileptics | Microsomal enzyme induction and high protein binding |
| *4. Antiplatelet drugs* | |
| Aspirin   } Dipyridamole | Delayed clotting |
| *5. Steroids* | Supplementation may be necessary because of adrenocortical suppression |
| *6. Eye drops* | |
| Phospholine iodide (Ecothiopate) | An anticholinesterase, prevents breakdown of suxamethonium |
| Timolol maleate | Systemic absorption causing bradycardia and bronchospasm |
| *7. Oral contraceptives* | See Chapter 3 |

Adapted from Shaw and Evans, 1988.

meaning of the term 'allergy' and may believe it refers to all adverse responses. For example, oversedation from benzodiazepines may be due to individual sensitivity or a relative overdose but can be described by a patient as an 'allergy', and the same applies to predictable side effects of some drugs such as itching, or nausea and vomiting. It is important to differentiate these unwanted but less serious effects from anaphylactoid syndromes.

A history of atopy does not identify patients at risk of anaphylaxis. However, patient's with a tendency to atopy may, when provoked, release histamine and other vasoactive substances, and may also have respiratory and cardiovascular systems that are more reactive when exposed to noxious stimuli.

The anaphylactoid (immediate) response to anaesthetic agents is an important cause of morbidity and mortality. Although severe reactions are rare, occurring once in every 5000–25 000 anaesthetics, they cause over 4% of anaesthetic deaths and nearly 6% of cases of cerebral damage (Noble and Yap, 1989). All anaesthetists should be able to recognize an anaphylactoid reaction and treat it vigorously and promptly. It has been suggested that an 'anaphylaxis drill' should be put into practice in this eventuality (Association of Anaesthetists, 1990) (Table 2.3).

**Table 2.3   Anaphylaxis drill, based on recommendations of the Association of Anaesthetists (1990)**

**Immediate management**
1.  Discontinue administration of suspect drug
2.  SUMMON HELP
3.  Discontinue surgery and anaesthesia if feasible
4.  Maintain airway with 100% oxygen. Intubation and ventilation will normally be indicated
5.  Give i.v. adrenaline 50–100 $\mu$g (0.5–1.0 ml 1:10 000). Further 1 ml aliquots as necessary
6.  Give i.v. volume, preferably colloid, 10 ml/kg rapidly
7.  Consider external chest compression

**Secondary management**
1.  For bronchospasm:
    salbutamol 250 $\mu$g i.v. then 5–20 $\mu$g min$^{-1}$ or terbutaline 250–500 $\mu$g i.v. then 1.5 $\mu$g min$^{-1}$ or aminophylline 6 $\mu$g kg$^{-1}$ i.v. over 20 min
2.  For bronchospasm and/or cardiovascular collapse:
    hydrocortisone 500 mg i.v. or methyl prednisolone 2 g i.v.
3.  Chlorpheniramine 20 mg i.v. diluted, given slowly
4.  Sodium bicarbonate if severe acidosis after 20 min of treatment
5.  Catecholamine infusions – adrenaline/noradrenaline
6.  Perform clotting screen
7.  Perform arterial blood gas analysis for oxygenation and acid-base status

All doses are for a 70 kg patient.
Basic monitoring is assumed.
Exercise caution if the diagnosis is not certain.

Estimates are that between 175 and 770 severe immediate drug reactions occur with general anaesthesia each year in the United Kingdom (Association of Anaesthetists, 1990). Certain drugs used in anaesthesia are particularly associated with adverse reactions (Watkins, 1989) (Table 2.4). The reported number of severe anaphylactoid reactions to a drug depends on the frequency with which it is used as well as its propensity to cause a reaction. Not surprisingly, thiopentone is the induction agent causing most reactions, with 68

reported in 1987 to the United Kingdom National Anaesthetic
Reactions Advisory Service, although 13 reactions were reported with
propofol, an agent which had only recently been introduced. Of the
muscle relaxants, suxamethonium causes most reactions and is undoubtedly the most hazardous of this group of drugs. Reactions to
local anaesthetics are very rare.

**Table 2.4   Anaesthetic agents ranked by reported number of severe anaphylactic reactions***

| Hypnotics | Muscle relaxants | Local anaesthetics |
|---|---|---|
| 1. Thiopentone | 1. Suxamethonium | 1. Bupivacaine |
| 2. Propofol | 2. Alcuronium | 2. Lignocaine |
| 3. Etomidate | 3. Atracurium | 3. Prilocaine |
| 4. Methohexitone | 4. Vecuronium | |
| | 5. Gallamine | |
| | 6. Tubocurarine | |
| | 7. Pancuronium | |

*As reported to UK National Adverse Anaesthetic Reactions Advisory Service in 1987. The
ranking reflects drug usage as well as frequency of reaction.

Some intravenous agents, of which morphine is an example, may
induce a pharmacological release of histamine but this rarely leads to
a life-threatening reaction. True anaphylaxis is associated with an IgE-
(or IgG-) mediated activation of inflammatory cells but nonim-
munological stimulation may lead to clinically indistinguishable
syndromes that are usually referred to as anaphylactoid reactions.
Identifying the precise cause of an allergic reaction is rarely easy at
the time of its occurrence, and the onset of severe symptoms may in
fact, be delayed for some time. Several drugs may have been administered within a short period and the anaesthetics may themselves
disguise the response so that cardiovascular collapse is often the first
noticeable manifestation of the reaction. Serial blood samples should
be taken in the first few hours for measurement of complement
activation, mast cell or basophil concentrations, and IgE or mediator
concentrations (Watkins, 1989). Although these tests may be helpful
in confirming that an anaphylactic reaction has occurred, they do not
help identify the causative agent.

If the patient survives the reaction, it is essential to attempt to
diagnose the precise trigger to avoid a further exposure, to recognize
that cross-sensitivity with other drugs may occur, and to communicate
the findings and stress their importance both to the patient and the
patient's general practitioner. The evaluation should start with a
detailed history of drug administration and previous allergic and
anaesthetic episodes (Weiss, Adkinson and Hirshman, 1989). Several

tests may be useful, including skin tests, basophil histamine release assays and radioallergosorbent tests (RAST). Intradermal skin testing a few weeks after a severe reaction will determine the drug responsible in 90% of cases. At present the RAST is available for only a limited number of anaesthetic drugs, including suxamethonium and thiopentone. The difficulty of interpretation, and the risks and expense of the tests do not make preoperative screening feasible at this time (Noble and Yap, 1989).

Although danger to life arises from the drugs administered during anaesthesia, it should not be forgotten that patients may be sensitive to other substances encountered during an anaesthetic. Sensitivity is usually manifested by contact with substances including adhesive tape, electrocardiogram skin electrodes, skin cleaning preparations, and even the rubber of face masks and other apparatus.

## Examination

### General examination

It is easy to suggest that a certain minimum examination is obligatory, but in common with other parts of the medical assessment it is important to weigh the amount of useful information gained against the time needed to obtain it. Thus the examiner needs to anticipate the chances of discovering an abnormality if one is present (sensitivity), and the chances of correctly identifying patients who have no abnormality (specificity). If an abnormality is discovered it must be decided whether the patient's perioperative management will be altered and what difference, if any, it will make to the outcome. There are no objective data available to assess this. Clearly if symptoms are present they will emerge when the history is taken and suggest to the examining doctor the required relevant examination. Although there are no published data, the authors would argue that there are very few asymptomatic findings that will profoundly affect the conduct of an anaesthetic. The common exceptions to this must include asymptomatic cardiac murmurs and severe hypertension. The airway should always be examined as a receding jaw, poor dentition and limited mouth opening do not produce significant symptoms but may profoundly affect the administration of an anaesthetic.

However there are further reasons for examining a patient carefully. The examination is safe for the patient and relatively cheap to perform. Even if there are no positive findings to record, the act of the physician 'laying on hands' and taking an interest in the patient has a reassuring and therapeutic effect, and will probably contribute towards relieving anxiety before an operation. The examination will also define the patient's preoperative status and is an opportunity to perform a 'health screen', even if it may not directly affect the conduct of the anaesthetic. Finally, the pre-anaesthetic examination is also useful to confirm and perhaps clarify the history, and they should therefore complement each other.

The examination as outlined in Table 2.5 is the minimum necessary to confirm symptoms and identify important unsuspected signs. The history, proposed operation and initial examination may suggest further examination and investigations needed in individual cases.

**Table 2.5    Suggested routine examination**

*General impression*    Overall wellbeing, weight, build, nutritional state, fluid state, colour of skin and mucous membranes to assess for anaemia, peripheral perfusion and jaundice. Measurement of temperature

*Cardiovascular system*    Pulse rate, volume and rhythm, blood pressure, cardiac impulses and heart sounds by auscultation, carotid pulsations, jugular venous pulsations, presence of sacral or ankle oedema

*Respiratory system*    Observe for dyspnoea, auscultate lungs

*Central nervous system*    Observe that the nervous system is grossly intact. The patient should be seen to move all four limbs, have normal hearing, vision and eye movements, and have no facial asymmetry

*Airway*    Mouth opening, neck flexion and extension, presence of dentures, loose teeth, crowns or bridgework

Further examination will be suggested by the history, the underlying pathology or the planned anaesthetic technique

There are some circumstances where even a brief examination may not be necessary, for example when the procedure is very minor, or where the patients are young and in perfect health. In these circumstances it can be argued that the likelihood of discovering an unsuspected and significant abnormality is very slight. To support this somewhat controversial viewpoint, we can only provide the evidence of many years of clinical practice in our paediatric general anaesthetic dental extraction service carried out on outpatients at the Dental School of the Royal London Hospital. Inhalational induction of anaesthesia is usually performed for procedures typically lasting less than 5 minutes. Preoperative assessment consists of a relevant history and, if this is normal, examination is restricted to an appreciation of the external appearance of the child including his or her vitality, skin and mucous membrane colour, and airway. Further examination is only performed when suggested by the history. This protocol has been followed for many years and there has been no evidence that patients have suffered preventable harm from it. In these and similar circumstances the practical and theoretical evidence does not support the necessity of a more thorough time-consuming examination as a routine. If it is intended to use local rather than general anaesthetic techniques, then the opinion expressed above is even more relevant.

## Preoperative assessment in selected conditions

There are several conditions which are associated with increased perioperative risk. The following list is not all-inclusive, but mentions the more important of these. An awareness and understanding of these problems can be used to direct the history, examination and investigations and to guide therapy to improve the patient's condition, as well as to provide information as to the anaesthetic requirements and the likely outcome from the anaesthetic and surgery.

### The 'difficult' airway

It is vital that the anaesthetist should be forewarned of patients who may present difficulty when maintaining a clear airway or intubating. This may be anticipated in patients with certain anatomical features such as a short, thick neck, protruding incisor teeth or a small, high arched palate. Further factors which can only be found by examination of the patient include inadequate flexion of the cervical spine with limited extension of the head at the atlanto-occipital joint, and difficulty in opening the mouth, either from immobility of the temporomandibular joint, or from trismus. Unfortunately a number of patients who on induction prove difficult to intubate present without obvious anatomical or pathological features at the initial anaesthetic assessment.

Much ingenuity has been expended to devise methods of reducing the number of unanticipated difficult intubations, for this would greatly enhance anaesthetic safety. One method of assessing potential difficulty is based on a four-point classification of pharyngeal structures seen when a patient opens the mouth wide and protrudes the tongue (Table 2.6) (Mallampati *et al.*, 1985). Difficulty in intubating may be anticipated in patients who fall into class III or IV (Samsoon and Young, 1987). The view at laryngoscopy has also been graded on a four-point scale with grades III and IV being associated with difficult intubation (Table 2.6) (Cormack and Lehane, 1984). Other techniques of varying usefulness have been described, including the angle subtended by various points on a lateral X-ray of head and neck (White and Kandor, 1975).

### Physical status

*ASA physical status*

The American Society of Anesthesiologists (ASA) classification may be used as a guide to the risks of anaesthesia (Vacanti, Van Houten

**Table 2.6    Methods of predicting a potentially difficult intubation based on a clinical assessment of pharyngeal and laryngeal anatomy**

1.  Pharyngeal structures seen with mouth open wide and tongue protruded (Mallampati *et al.*, 1985)

    Class I:    soft palate, fauces, uvula and pillars
    Class II:   soft palate, fauces, uvula
    Class III:  soft palate, base of uvula
    Class IV:   soft palate not visible at all

2.  View at laryngoscopy (Cormack and Lehane, 1984)

    Grade I:    full view of glottis
    Grade II:   only posterior commissure visible
    Grade III:  only tip of epiglottis visible
    Grade IV:   no glottic structure visible

and Hill, 1970: Lewin *et al.*, 1971; Cohen and Duncan, 1988). Patients are divided into five classes based on their general health, and each category is modified by whether the surgery contemplated is performed electively or as an emergency. Further details are given in Table 2.7. Although intraoperative complication rates increase with increasing ASA status and with surgery performed as an emergency (Hudson *et al.*, 1990), this classification is nonspecific, poorly predictive of outcome and gives no help in identifying ways in which risk can be decreased.

**Table 2.7    American Society of Anesthesiologists (ASA) physical status measure**

*Class I*    There is no physiologic, biochemical, or psychiatric disturbance. The pathological process for which the operation is to be performed is localized and not conducive to systemic disturbance. Examples: a fit patient with inguinal hernia; fibroid uterus in otherwise healthy woman

*Class II*    Mild to moderate systemic disturbance caused either by the condition to be treated surgically or other pathophysiological processes. Examples: mild diabetes, essential hypertension, or anaemia

*Class III*    Rather severe systemic disturbance of pathology from whatever cause, even though it may not be possible to define the degree of disability with finality. Examples: severe diabetes with vascular complications; moderate to severe degrees of pulmonary insufficiency; angina or healed myocardial infarction

*Class IV*    Indicative of the patient with a severe systemic disorder already life-threatening and not always correctable by the operative procedure. Examples: advanced degrees of cardiac, pulmonary, hepatic, renal or endocrine insufficiency

*Class V*    The moribund patient who has little chance of survival. Examples: the burst abdominal aneurysm in a patient with profound shock; major cerebral trauma with rapidly increasing intracranial pressure; massive pulmonary embolus

*Emergency operation (E)*    Any patient in one of the classes listed above who is operated upon as an emergency

*Obesity*

Obesity is associated with increased risks under anaesthesia and in the postoperative period (Fox, Whalley and Bevan, 1981; Fisher, Waterhouse and Adams, 1975). Patients who are 30% overweight have a 40% increased chance of dying from heart disease and a 50% increased risk of a stroke. Obese people have cardiac and pulmonary abnormalities, they present airway and other technical challenges, are at increased risk of aspiration, and may handle drugs in an abnormal way. Obese patients may resort to drastic dieting or surgery such as intestinal tract bypass operations in an attempt to conquer their problem and this in turn may produce metabolic and electrolyte abnormalities.

## Cardiovascular system

### Cardiac risk factors

Goldman and co-authors (1977) described risk factors which identify the potential for cardiac problems in patients undergoing noncardiac surgery. These are listed in Table 2.8. Patients are awarded points for risk factors to a total score of 53. The most important risk factors are cardiac failure, a recent myocardial infarction and serious abnormalities of cardiac rhythm. The risk associated with cardiac failure is confirmed by others (Driksen and Thomas, 1988) and failure must be controlled before surgery. A Cardiac Risk Index score of more than 13 carries increased risks of cardiac morbidity and mortality, and with a score of more than 26 it has been recommended that only truly life-saving surgery should be considered. Although severe cardiac illness is undoubtedly associated with an increase in perioperative morbidity and mortality, since the study of Goldman was performed there have been considerable advances in the understanding and treatment of cardiac pathology, and this is likely to be reflected in a better outcome after surgery in these patients.

**Table 2.8   The Goldman Cardiac Risk Index**

| Criteria | Points |
| --- | --- |
| Cardiac failure (S3, gallop, raised JVP) | 11 |
| MI in previous 6 months | 10 |
| Rhythm other than sinus or premature atrial contractions | 7 |
| Five premature ventricular contractions/min at any time preoperatively | 7 |
| Age > 70 years | 5 |
| Emergency | 4 |
| Important valvular aortic stenosis | 3 |
| Abnormal blood gases, electrolytes, bed-ridden or chronic liver disease | 3 |
| Operation: intraperitoneal, intrathoracic, aortic | 3 |
| Total | 53 |

Based on Goldman *et al.* (1977).

## Previous myocardial infarction

A recent myocardial infarction increases the risk of reinfarction in the perioperative period. The risks are much higher within 6 months of an infarct but are probably also related to the residual effects of the infarct. The risks of the anaesthetic must be balanced against the urgency of the surgery and, whenever possible, surgery should be delayed. Putting off the surgery for only 1 or 2 months may be of benefit but ideally the delay should be for 6 months or preferably 1 year after the infarct. If the operation cannot be delayed, precise haemodynamic control and postoperative monitoring in an Intensive Care Unit have been shown to decrease mortality (Rao, Jacobs and El-Etr, 1983).

## Ischaemic heart disease

Although evidence for the anaesthetic risk in patients suffering from angina is not as clear-cut as in those who have had a previous myocardial infarction, the anaesthetic technique has been shown to affect the chances of precipitating perioperative ischaemia in patients at risk, and the incidence of postoperative myocardial infarction is related, at least in part, to the number of perioperative ischaemic episodes (Slogoff and Keats, 1985). Angina is an especially important symptom as it may be the only indicator of the ischaemic heart disease. The New York Heart Association Classification of Angina (Table 2.9) is a simple clinical classification that is commonly used to grade the severity of ischaemic heart disease. There are four grades of activity, from grade I, where angina is only brought on by strenuous activity, to grade IV, where angina may be present at rest.

Table 2.9   New York Heart Association Classification of Angina

---

*Grade I*   No limitation of ordinary physical activity, e.g. walking or climbing stairs does not cause angina. Angina is caused by strenuous or rapid prolonged exertion at work or recreation or with sexual relations

*Grade II*   Slight limitation of normal activity, e.g. walking or climbing stairs rapidly, walking uphill, walking or stair climbing after meals, or in cold, or in wind, or under emotional stress, or only during a few hours after awakening

*Grade III*   Marked limitation of ordinary physical activity, e.g. after walking one or two blocks on the level or climbing one flight of stairs. 'Comfortable at rest'

*Grade IV*   Inability to carry on any physical activity without discomfort, e.g. angina may be present at rest

---

## Hypertension

Hypertension is associated in the long term with an increased risk of stroke, cardiac disease and renal insufficiency. Epidemiological studies have suggested that patients with a diastolic blood pressure greater than 90 mmHg should be treated with antihypertensives. Although the evidence is not conclusive, untreated hypertension is also probably associated with an increased mortality under anaesthesia (Asiddao, 1982), and systolic hypertension may increase postoperative morbidity and the lability of the blood pressure under anaesthesia (Bedford and Feinstein, 1980). It has also been suggested that the level above which anaesthetic risk increases is a diastolic blood pressure of 110 mmHg and that this may be more important than the level of systolic blood pressure. Individual preoperative values should be noted and in-traoperative management directed towards maintaining cardiovascular variables within this range. Consideration should be given to administering a beta-blocking drug as part of the premedication. It is not always easy to measure preoperative blood pressure accurately as patients are often nervous and may show an anxiety-related rise in blood pressure, the so-called 'white coat hypertension'. If the diastolic blood pressure is above 110 mmHg repeat measurements should be made with the patient confined to bed, and charted for a period of several hours. The use of an automatic noninvasive machine to measure blood pressure may provide more accurate measurements.

### Valvular heart disease

The nature of the valvular heart disease must be ascertained. Management of stenotic or regurgitant lesions of the same valve are different and associated cardiac failure or ischaemia may be present. There are increased risks of dysrhythmias, emboli and endocarditis. Anticoagulation may be necessary and must be carefully controlled in the perioperative period. Antibiotic cover will be required.

### Conduction disorders

Premature ventricular contractions, premature atrial contractions and rhythms other than sinus are associated with increased risk, probably because the conduction defects reflect an underlying cardiac disorder. A pacemaker-dependent patient will not be able to increase the heart rate to boost cardiac output and will therefore need especially careful control of intravascular volume during procedures involving large fluid shifts or changes in systemic vascular resistance. The pacemaker may also be affected by diathermy and this must be determined for the specific pacemaker, which if necessary can usually be converted with a magnet to fixed rate pacing.

## Respiratory system

### Asthma

Asthmatics have irritable airways and may develop bronchospasm in response to anaesthetic drugs or from physical stimuli such as laryngoscopy or intubation. The patients must be on optimal medical therapy and elective procedures should not take place unless their condition is as good as possible. Prophylaxis against an attack and the use of antibiotics and physiotherapy may be useful and this is discussed further in Chapter 3.

### Chronic obstructive pulmonary disease

Chronic bronchitis is said to be present when a patient has a history of a chronic productive cough on most days for more than three months for at least two successive years. The potential anaesthetic problems are related to the increased risk of infection and atelectasis, the element of reversible airways disease that may be present, and hypoxic ventilatory drive that can make some patients unresponsive to the respiratory stimulus of carbon dioxide. An assessment is necessary to ascertain whether therapy with antibiotics, bronchodilators and physiotherapy is indicated. Care must be taken when administering oxygen as high concentrations may depress respiration.

## Nervous system

Some anaesthetic agents, including enflurane and methohexitone, are epileptogenic and should be avoided in patients with epilepsy. Special anaesthetic considerations are necessary for patients with raised intracranial pressure and these are described in any textbook of neurosurgical anaesthesia. If the patient has a disease that causes a neurological deficit it is wise to describe the extent of the deficit carefully and to indicate the rate of progression at the preoperative assessment. Although there is no evidence to suggest that regional anaesthesia exacerbates such conditions, if there is a deterioration in the patient's neurological condition during the postoperative period the use of local anaesthetics may delay the discovery of such a deficit and be blamed by the patient, or even some physicians, for the changes.

## Gastrointestinal and liver disease

### Increased risk of aspiration

Many prepared patients for elective surgery have significant volumes of acid secretions in their stomachs but fortunately appear to have little risk of aspirating these gastric contents. There are some patients, however, who have an increased risk of aspiration. These include those who have recently eaten, are in pain, have been the victims of trauma and are receiving opiates. A history of hiatus hernia or anything that increases intragastric pressure or decreases gastro-oesophageal sphincter pressures – such as obesity or pregnancy – will also increase the risk, as will conditions which depress protective airway reflexes.

*Liver disease*

A patient with liver disease may have metabolic derangement, central nervous system toxicity, coagulation abnormalities, cardiac and respiratory dysfunction, nutritional disorders and an increased risk of renal failure and sepsis. Anaesthesia in such patients is associated with an increased risk of morbidity and mortality.

Although anaesthetic agents, such as halothane, may transiently adversely affect the results of liver function tests, hypoxia, hypoperfusion, sepsis and trauma may be more important in this respect. The rare, and often fatal, severe hepatic necrosis associated with the use of halothane should be considered separately and here medico-legal considerations may affect the choice of inhalational agent. The possibility of hepatitis B must be considered as must the risk of HIV, especially in intravenous drugs abusers, and staff must be particularly assiduous when protecting themselves from contamination with the patient's blood or saliva.

## Renal disease

Patients with renal disease present difficulties with fluid and electrolyte management. Uraemia has many systemic manifestations and may affect the cardiovascular, pulmonary, immunological, haematological and nervous systems. Conditions associated with renal failure include cardiac failure, hypertension, anaemia and diabetes. Acute renal failure developing in the perioperative period is associated with increased mortality and the anaesthetist must do everything possible to preserve renal function in patients at risk. In assessing patients with established renal failure it is important to ascertain when the most recent dialysis was performed and care must be taken to preserve the integrity of the venous access site in the case of haemodialysis or the peritoneal catheter for peritoneal dialysis. Arrangements need to be made to maintain the dialysis in the perioperative period.

Many drugs are excreted, at least to some extent, by the renal route and this will influence the agents chosen and the amounts used. Drugs that are potentially nephrotoxic must be avoided. In appropriate patients mannitol, diuretics and renal vasodilators, along with appropriate fluid therapy, may have a role in maintaining renal function.

## Metabolic and endocrine disorders

*Diabetes mellitus*

A patient with diabetes has an increased likelihood of having associated cardiac, renal and cerebral atherosclerotic disease, peripheral neuropathies and autonomic dysfunction. In the post-operative period infection and impaired wound healing are possibilities. Diabetics are also subject to the risks of hypoglycaemia from an overdose of insulin, and ketoacidosis and hyperosmolar states from poor control of blood sugar. Abnormalities should be sought in those systems known to be affected by diabetes, and treatment should be optimized preoperatively. Many regimes have been suggested for the perioperative control of blood glucose (Hirsch *et al.*, 1991) and, although the evidence does not clearly demonstrate a decreased incidence of postoperative complications in patients in whom the blood sugar is controlled within tight limits, until there is evidence to the contrary the aim of the physician must be to achieve such control.

## Adrenal cortical malfunction

Glucocorticoids, mineralocorticoids and androgens are secreted by the adrenal cortex. Excess secretion of androgens causes no specific problems related to anaesthesia.

Cushing's syndrome is caused by an excess secretion of glucocorticoids and is associated with thin, easily bruised skin and difficulty gaining peripheral venous access, osteoporosis, hypertension, fluid retention and sometimes a proximal myopathy or diabetes mellitus. One cause is exogenous steroid therapy and this may cause adrenocortical suppression requiring replacement steroid therapy during the perioperative period. This topic is discussed in Chapter 3. If the increased secretion of glucocorticoids is secondary to an ACTH-producing tumour or a primary adrenal tumour, then preoperative treatment should be primarily directed at the effect of the steroid on the end organs by managing the resulting hypertension and disorders of fluids and electrolytes.

Adrenal cortical insufficiency may be secondary to defects in ACTH secretion or from destruction or suppression of the adrenal gland. If patients with this condition are stressed they may experience an acute adrenal crisis (Addisonian crisis) resulting in cardiovascular collapse. They are likely to be dehydrated, anaemic and debilitated, and preoperative preparation should be directed towards correcting any hypovolaemia and electrolyte abnormalities. They will need adequate steroid therapy (300 mg 70 $kg^{-1}$ $day^{-1}$) to cover the perioperative period.

Excess mineralocorticoid secretion (Conn's syndrome) leads to symptoms associated with hyperaldosteronism. The retention of sodium expands the blood volume and causes hypertension, while hypokalaemia is associated with weakness, alkalosis and sometimes nephropathy. Treatment is with spironolactone with attention to intravascular fluid volume, correction of electrolytes and renal function.

*Abnormalities of thyroid function*

An overactive thyroid will give rise to a patient history of weight loss, diarrhoea, irritability, restlessness and insomnia. Examination may reveal an enlarged thyroid, exophthalmos, tachycardia, ventricular ectopic beats and other cardiac dysrhythmias, heart failure and muscle weakness. Its most dramatic manifestation is a 'thyroid storm' or thyrotoxic crisis with fever, cardiac dysrhythmias and collapse. Emergency treatment is symptomatic with B-adrenergic blockade and sedation followed by antithyroid medication.

A patient with hypothyroidism will be lethargic, somnolent, constipated and intolerant of the cold. Physical signs include a bradycardia, heart failure and pericardial and pleural effusions. Preoperative management consists of administering thyroid hormones to attain normal thyroid function and, in an emergency, supportive therapy to restore intravascular volume, electrolyte balance, and cardiac and respiratory function.

*Excess secretion of growth hormone (acromegaly)*

Excessive growth hormone results in bony deformities and an increase in connective tissue, both of which may complicate airway management and make endotracheal intubation difficult. There is an enlargement of all the organs of the body. Hypertension is common and in some patients cardiomyopathy develops which may lead to cardiac failure. Respiratory function is often impaired because of kyphoscoliosis, and renal function may also be diminished. Diabetes mellitus is also possible, as are fluid and electrolyte abnormalities. Preoperative assessment and management is directed towards the airway and significant cardiac, respiratory or diabetic problems.

## Neuromuscular disorders

*Neuropathies and myopathies*

Neuropathies and myopathies may be associated with abnormalities of respiratory and sometimes cardiac function. Several of the drugs used during anaesthesia have to be avoided or used with care, and this especially includes the use of muscle relaxants.

*Malignant hyperthermia*

Malignant hyperthermia is a muscle disorder that results in severe metabolic abnormalities and is usually associated with extreme elevation in body temperature (Gronert, 1980). It results from a defect on chromosome 19 and is transferred as an autosomal dominant trait with variable expressivity and reportedly has an incidence of 1 : 15 000 anaesthetics in children and 1:50000 in adults. Almost all episodes are triggered by agents used only in anaesthesia and these include all the potent inhalational anaesthetics and the depolarizing muscle relaxant suxamethonium. Atropine, digoxin and anticholinesterase agents should also be avoided as there is evidence that they can trigger or exacerbate the reaction.

If an episode of malignant hyperthermia remains unrecognized mortality is high, and it is therefore important to consider the possibility when taking the patient or family history, or administering an anaesthetic (Hackl *et al.*, 1990). Malignant hyperthermia is associated with other muscular disorders including strabismus, muscle cramps, scoliosis, Duchenne's muscular dystrophy, myotonia congenita and osteogenesis imperfecta. Previous uneventful anaesthetics do not confirm that the patient is not susceptible, as exposure to precipitating agents will not always trigger the syndrome in a given individual. A family history of unexplained sudden anaesthetic deaths is suggestive and should be explored further. Diagnosis requires a muscle biopsy.

The early symptoms include trismus after suxamethonium, although this is not a helpful sign as it may frequently occur without leading to malignant hyperthermia, sudden unexplained tachycardia or arrhythmia, skeletal muscle rigidity, unstable blood pressure, tachypnoea, cyanosis, hypercarbia and metabolic acidosis. Although the increase in temperature is of diagnostic importance, it will usually follow these other manifestations.

If malignant hyperthermia is suspected, anaesthetic management will include the use of a vapour-free anaesthetic machine and a regional or general anaesthetic technique that avoids the use of triggering agents. Extensive monitoring will be necessary during the anaesthetic and recovery periods. Dantrolene sodium is a directly acting skeletal muscle relaxant and can help in the prophylaxis and treatment of this condition. If an episode of malignant hyperthermia occurs in an anaesthetized patient the anaesthetic and surgery should be stopped if at all possible, or if not a 'safe' anaesthetic technique adopted. The patient should be actively cooled and the acidosis and metabolic abnormalities must be corrected. The minimum essential monitoring is of the electrocardiogram, oxygen saturation, temperature (core and peripheral), urinary output and arterial and central venous pressures. Intravenous dantrolene (2.5 mg kg$^{-1}$ repeated up to 10 mg kg$^{-1}$) must be administered and supportive therapy given as indicated to support vital organ function.

## Psychiatric conditions

The patient with psychiatric problems may react to the prospect of anaesthesia and surgery in an emotional or unusual manner. Careful repeated explanation and reassurance may be needed and the anaesthetist should be especially sensitive to the wishes and fears of the patient. The patient may be taking mood altering drugs such as monoamine oxidase inhibitors (MAOI) and tricyclic antidepressants. MAOIs may cause severe hypertension with indirectly acting sympathetic drugs such as ephedrine. Convulsions, hyperpyrexia and coma have occasionally been reported with some opioids, particularly pethidine which must be avoided. Conventional wisdom has been to discontinue MAOIs several weeks before anaesthesia but this is not universally accepted as necessary. Tricyclic antidepressants block adrenergic re-uptake into the cells and enhance the action of directly acting catecholamines. They often have atropine-like actions and can cause arrhythmias, especially with an anaesthetic which includes halothane and pancuronium.

Patients who are having a course of electroconvulsive therapy (ECT) will require several anaesthetics over a short time period. The ECT usually triggers a sudden massive increase in blood pressure which may on occasion result in intracerebral haemorrhage or myocardial ischaemia. Although the anaesthesia for ECT is brief these patients need a complete relevant assessment and those at risk will require careful monitoring and control of blood pressure during the procedure.

# Investigations

Investigations in the laboratory or X-ray and imaging department are essential elements in diagnosis. They are necessary to discover or quantify abnormalities before a diagnosis can be confirmed, and in anaesthetic practice they are often used to establish baseline values. Rarely investigations may be used as screening tests for abnormalities which would profoundly affect the conduct of an anaesthetic. An example of this would be screening for sickle cell disease or trait. Extensive routine testing in patients with a normal history and examination is unlikely to produce results that would affect anaesthetic management or its outcome.

In deciding whether a test is worthwhile, the person requesting it must anticipate the probable result, and the effect this would have on the anaesthetic. In relation to pre-anaesthetic assessment, a test is only worth performing if an abnormal result would affect the anaesthetic management, and there appear to be few situations where this is so if the result is not anticipated by the history and examination. In many instances abnormal results are apparently ignored by the doctors and the procedure goes ahead with no adverse effects. This either indicates that desirable treatment is not given, or more likely that unnecessary tests are performed. If important abnormalities are discovered appropriate treatment, if indicated, must be carried out before the operation.

No invasive procedure is free of risk, including the physical risk of radiation from X-rays or the possibility of injury or infection from needles. A proportion of the tests will give a false positive result which can increase patient anxiety and may delay surgery. Further physical morbidity may occur if other investigations are needed and performed, especially if they are of increasing complexity. Finally the cost of performing the test should be considered, as this is not inconsiderable and will be wasted if the test does not contribute useful information relevant to the wellbeing of the anaesthetized patient.

# General considerations

## Normal values

Normal values are derived from testing a large number of apparently healthy people and will vary from laboratory to laboratory. To define the normal range of haemoglobin the values are measured in a sample, say of 1000 volunteers. This will produce a range of values, and the normal range is commonly defined as values between the 2.5th percentile and the 97.5th percentile. This defines as 'abnormal' the lowest and the highest 2.5%. The limitations are obvious when we see that of the 1000 million population in China 50 million will statistically be defined as having abnormal values of haemoglobin! In the same way when multiple tests are performed the likelihood of an abnormal result arising by chance increases. If a battery of 15 tests is performed then statistically over half the patients are likely to have at least one abnormal result (Bradwell *et al.*, 1974). The sample used to determine a normal range may also present shortcomings, for example British medical students commonly used in determining normal physiological values may not be appropriate for the Chinese population.

A high proportion of healthy patients with initially 'abnormal' results will be found to have values within the normal range on retesting. Accurate measurements depend on the proper maintenance and use of laboratory equipment, with trained staff and proper quality control methods. Any lapse in the standards will increase the chance of unusual or abnormal results, and therefore the results of any test must be interpreted with careful consideration of the applicability to the particular individual. Only when the history, examination and investigations reinforce each other do they become significant.

## Preoperative tests to screen for abnormalities

Most investigations should be initiated after discovery of abnormalities from the history or examination, or to establish preoperative baseline values. A list of conditions that can be picked up by preoperative screening which may affect surgical outcome or procedures has been suggested (Robbins and Mushlin, 1979; Roizen, 1986) (Table 2.10). It should be noted that few patients with these abnormalities would be asymptomatic, and most of the relevant investigations are not usually performed preoperatively, with several of them requiring special expertise or invasive techniques. A test that is useful as a screen for abnormalities should, in modern Western medicine, be applied to the population at large and not just those who happen to turn up for an operation.

**Table 2.10   Important conditions detected by laboratory testing**

1. Cardiac: ischaemic heart disease, cardiac dysrhythmias, congestive heart failure
2. Respiratory: chronic obstructive pulmonary disease, chronic interstitial lung disease
3. Endocrine: diabetes, thyroid disease, phaeochromocytoma, Addison's disease, Cushing's disease, inappropriate antidiuretic hormone (ADH) secretion
4. Haematological: anaemia, thrombocytopenia, clotting disorders, haemoglobinopathies
5. Infectious: hepatitis, syphilis, tuberculosis, urinary tract infection, gonorrhoea, HIV infection
6. Renal: nephrotic syndrome, nephritis
7. Miscellaneous: glaucoma, increased intracranial pressure, pregnancy

Investigations are most useful when applied to a selected population with a high chance of demonstrating an abnormality, rather than the population at large. Therefore tests should be restricted to those with a reasonable likelihood of having an abnormality. A simple questionnaire has been shown to be effective in selecting patients who require a full blood count, coagulation screen, urea and electrolytes, liver function test and electrocardiogram (ECG). In particular, if the specific indication has to be stated by the requesting doctor before a test is performed it has been estimated that a cost saving of 50% or more could be achieved (Roizen, 1986). The frequency of preoperative X-rays could also be reduced by half for the same reasons with no apparent increase in morbidity or mortality (Fowkes et al., 1986).

*Ward-based laboratories*

Small, user-friendly, relatively inexpensive machines are now available to perform a variety of investigations on the ward. Apparatus is available to give results including haemoglobin, sodium, potassium, calcium, glucose, urea, albumin, lactate, arterial blood gases, oxygen saturation, carboxyhaemoglobin and methaemoglobin. Although there are advantages in terms of accessibility and speed of result (Marks, 1983), problems exist with operator training and quality control. Unless equipment is properly maintained and samples are correctly taken and measured, the accuracy of the results cannot be relied upon (Verma, Dhond and Lawler, 1990). Furthermore, a record of the results and the time of measurement may not always be put in the notes to be available for later consideration.

### Batch analysis

Many investigations are cheaper when the laboratory is able to perform similar tests in batches, and repeat them at infrequent intervals. The laboratory would usually prefer to receive a relatively large number of samples to analyse at one time rather than fewer samples scattered over the working day or week. Many tests are now performed by autoanalysers that will report a large list of results on a single sample even if only one test is required by the clinician. In addition, unnecessary tests are sometimes ordered by the doctor because it is often not possible to take a full history and perform an examination to decide which tests are indicated before the laboratory needs the samples. Earlier preoperative assessment, perhaps in a clinic or by means of a questionnaire, would avoid this dilemma and also save costs.

## The result of the investigation

If a test is ordered it must be presumed that the result is of importance in determining the treatment of the patient concerned. Therefore the results must be obtained and considered by those concerned before the operation is due to start, all of which may require considerable organization and effort. Unfortunately many results are not examined or appropriately followed up in advance of surgery, and this may not only put a patient at risk but also has medico-legal implications if a mishap arises. For these reasons, as well as the waste of resources from unnecessary testing, only investigations that are indicated should be requested.

## Indications for investigations

Investigations are indicated in the following patients:

### Where there are pre-existing medical conditions

This is to provide baseline values and to guide the anaesthetist as to whether preoperative treatment is indicated. The exact test depends on the specific pathology, medication taken and likely interreactions during the anaesthetic.

## When major surgery is contemplated

In these circumstances baseline values of various parameters are desirable, for example haemoglobin, urea and electrolytes and liver function tests. Where medical personnel may be at risk from contact with the patient's blood, for example with procedures such as cardiac surgery, a screen for hepatitis B is often performed. At present there is debate over whether such a screen should be extended to patients from groups with a high incidence of HIV infection. Infection with the virus profoundly affects a patient's life, including sexual and social relationships, employment and insurance prospects, and the impact of a positive test must be weighed against the potential risk to hospital staff. In the view of the authors, it would seem reasonable that hospital staff should be able to confirm the presence of the disease before operating upon such high-risk patients.

## Selection for investigation

It is possible to select for special investigation subgroups of patients who are likely to have a higher than normal chance of having an abnormality. For example, the routine chest X-ray would reveal about 1.5% of new abnormalities in the under-40 age group, but up to 30% in the over-60s. Again the prevalence of electrocardiographic abnormalities increases from 10% at 35 years to 25% by the age of 57, and the incidence of ischaemic heart disease, renal and hepatic diseases also increases with age. The sex of the patient may determine the need for investigation, and examples are the higher incidence of anaemia in menstruating females, and ischaemic heart disease at a younger age in males.

Based on the available information, we have made suggestions for a system of screening tests that could be applied to asymptomatic healthy patients about to undergo body surface procedures with minimal blood loss (Table 2.11). Needless to say, these guidelines cannot cover all contingencies and the clinical judgement of the patient's doctor should always be the final guide to the need for investigations.

Table 2.11   Guidelines for investigation in asymptomatic healthy patients

| Age (yr) | Male | Female |
| --- | --- | --- |
| Under 40 | None | Haemoglobin only |
| 40–60 | Haemoglobin | Haemoglobin |
| | Urea and electrolytes | Urea and electrolytes |
| | ECG | |
| Over 60 | Haemoglobin | Haemoglobin |
| | Glucose | Glucose |
| | Urea and electrolytes | Urea and electrolytes |
| | ECG | ECG |
| | Chest X-ray | Chest X-ray |

## Routine preoperative tests

### Full blood count

Uncontrolled polycythaemia (haemoglobin > 16 g/dl) is associated with an increased incidence of complications, including haemorrhage and thrombosis, and is therefore a risk factor for patients undergoing major surgery. Mild anaemia is probably not harmful, but arbitrary values of haemoglobin (e.g. 9.0 g $dl^{-1}$) are usually accepted as the lower limit for patients undergoing minor procedures or elective surgery where blood loss is not anticipated. Because of physiological adjustments, chronic anaemia is tolerated better than an acute drop in haemoglobin, and patients with a poor coronary circulation or limited cardiac or respiratory reserve will be more at risk than others from acute anaemia. Anaemia is associated with many diseases that may affect anaesthetic management, including renal insufficiency or a drug reaction, and if a patient is discovered to be anaemic a cause should be sought. It is rare to discover abnormal results in asymptomatic patients. Of 2117 routine preoperative haemoglobin results for patients undergoing oral and maxillofacial surgery, only seven, all from females, were unexpectedly found to be less than 10 g $dl^{-1}$ (Walton, 1988).

### Blood chemistry

This includes the measurement of urea, creatinine and electrolytes, liver function tests and plasma glucose. Unexpected findings with screening are discovered in less than 1% of patients under the age of 40 (Campbell and Gosling, 1988). The incidence of abnormalities of urea and electrolyte measurement increases with age (McKee and Scott, 1987) and with ASA grade (McCleane, 1988), being approximately 50% for those over 60 years of age or ASA grade IV or V. Although abnormal findings often lead to further investigations, in about 80% of the cases the results do not affect patient management. Most abnormalities are of blood glucose and urea. In modern laboratories, requesting one test will produce an array of other results. For some tests (e.g. calcium), the false positive rate is so high that the test is valueless. A problem of what action to take may arise when a test, not requested, is reported to be abnormal.

### Chest X-ray

About 4% of routine preoperative chest X-rays will detect an abnormality (Royal College Working Party, 1979) but this incidence will be less in patients under 40 years of age. Few of these abnormalities are unsuspected after taking a history and performing an examination, and most of the abnormalities are unlikely to affect treatment. There is little evidence to support the need for a baseline preoperative X-ray against which subsequent radiographs showing postoperative pulmonary complications can be judged. The incidence of false positives with conditions such as pneumonia is such that when screening large numbers of patients almost as many will be falsely diagnosed positive as those who actually have the disease (Tape and Mushlin, 1986). A routine X-ray will therefore not only be useless for healthy patients but may prove harmful if an abnormality leads to further investigations which may include bronchoscopy or even thoracotomy. Screening for disease with chest X-rays should therefore be reserved for populations at high risk of an abnormality, and radiographs should only be requested in patients under 60 years of age if there is a clear indication. A list of indications for ordering a preoperative chest X-ray is given in Table 2.12.

**Table 2.12  Indications for requesting a preoperative chest X-ray**

1. History of active lung disease
2. Physical signs of active lung disease
3. Symptoms and signs of heart disease
4. Over 60 years of age
5. Intrathoracic surgery
6. History of smoking, exposure to asbestos
7. Cancer at any site
8. Abdominal tenderness, organomegaly or ascites
9. Recent immigrants from countries where tuberculosis is still endemic who have not had a chest X-ray within the previous 12 months

Adapted from Dresner and Soni (1989).

*Electrocardiogram (ECG)*

Various abnormalities may be detected by a 12-lead electrocardiogram including alterations in rhythm, ischaemic changes and indications of previous myocardial infarction (Goldberger and O'Konski, 1986). Many of these ECG changes should be suspected from the history or examination. These changes are important as there is an increased morbidity and mortality from recent infarction, left ventricular hypertrophy and ventricular extrasystoles and in many cases preoperative treatment or postponement of the operation may be of benefit to the patient. The resting ECG may not uncover important disease, as it is normal in up to 50% of patients with coronary artery disease. The ECG is an inefficient means of detecting cardiac abnormalities unless the population selected for testing has a high prevalence of abnormal findings (Rabkin and Horne, 1983). A list of indications for ordering a preoperative ECG is given in Table 12.13.

*Urinalysis*

This test has the advantage of being noninvasive, easy to perform and

Table 2.13    **Recommendations for preoperative electrocardiograms (ECG)**

---

1. Patients with history of heart disease
2. Patients with physical signs of heart disease
3. Men aged over 40 years
4. Women aged over 55 years
5. Systemic disease associated with cardiac involvement, e.g. hypertension, peripheral vascular disease, diabetes mellitus, collagen vascular diseases, rheumatic fever
6. Patients on potentially cardiotoxic drugs
7. Surgery associated with cardiac complications
8. Patients at risk of major electrolyte abnormalities

---

Adapted from Dresner, 1989.

relatively cheap. The finding of protein or glucose is a screen for renal disease or diabetes. However, as a screening test the number of false positives is about twice as great as with blood biochemistry and published data do not support the efficacy of routine preoperative urinalysis (Lawrence and Kroenke, 1988).

## Further investigations

Certain specific investigations are required in some patients, and when indicated the following investigations may be essential before operation.

### Testing for sickle cell disease and thalassaemia

A number of genotypes are associated with *in vivo* sickling of red cells (Davies and Brozovic, 1989). These include haemoglobin HbSS (sickle cell disease), HbAS (sickle cell trait) and HbSC. In the United States and the United Kingdom the prevalence of the HbS gene is about 10% of the black population. The homozygous state is correspondingly rarer. Haemoglobin C disease has a prevalence of about 2% in British and American blacks. Patients with sickle cell disease are almost always severely affected by their disease, with bony deformities, clinical anaemia and mild jaundice. Myocardial fibrosis may cause cardiac dysfunction and in adults the spleen may be small and fibrotic from multiple splenic infarcts. In contrast, patients with sickle cell trait are usually clinically normal. Screening for sickle cell disease should be carried out in patients at risk of carrying the gene. The Sickledex test, which relies on the insolubility of HbS, is a quick screening test but, if positive, must be followed by haemoglobin electrophoresis to identify the genotype. Preoperative preparation of a patient with sickle cell disease may require exchange transfusion. Published reports indicate that the complications of anaesthesia in patients with haemoglobinopathies are uncommon provided hypoxia can be avoided (Sears, 1978; Homi *et al.*, 1979).

It should be noted that another cause of anaemia, glucose-6-phosphate dehydrogenase (G6-PD) deficiency, is widespread in populations where the sickle gene is prevalent. This defect is associated with red cell haemolysis after administration of drugs that produce substances requiring G6-PD for detoxification.

In thalassaemia there is a deficiency in the production of either the alpha or beta haemoglobin chain and abnormal tetramers are produced which may precipitate and damage the red cell. The presentation is similar in many ways to that of sickle cell disorders in that the homozygous individuals may have life-shortening anaemia whilst those who are heterozygote often have no symptoms. Thalassaemia is found over a wide region, including those countries surrounding the Mediterranean Sea. Diagnosis is made from a positive family history confirmed by examination of a blood film and haemoglobin electrophoresis.

## Clotting studies

There appears to be no place for routine clotting studies in all patients, but these investigations should be reserved for when there is a suspicion of abnormal coagulation, something which is often suggested by the history (Rohrer, Michelotti and Nahrwold, 1988). Examples are a patient with hepatic or renal dysfunction, or a story of abnormal bleeding or bruising.

Disorders of platelet function are commonly drug-related, although they may be secondary to immune disease or rarely an inherited defect. The drug-related defects are ones of platelet aggregation and release caused by an effect on platelet cyclo-oxygenase. Clinical presentation is with a history of bleeding of the skin or mucosa, and platelet function should be assessed with a whole blood bleeding test.

## Respiratory function tests

Although pulmonary complications are a common and an important cause of postoperative morbidity, respiratory function tests are generally not helpful in predicting the patients likely to suffer this postoperative complication. In particular spirometry appears to add little to clinical information, does not uncover relevant hidden disease and has no effect on individual patient outcome (Lawrence, Page and Harris, 1989). A patient's arterial blood gases, particularly the $Pao_2$, along with a clinical assessment of the degree of dyspnoea, do provide a guide to the necessity of postoperative ventilation (Nunn et al., 1988). Pulmonary function tests are essential to provide baseline measurements for patients about to undergo lung resection, although practical tests of exercise tolerance, such as walking up stairs, are also of value.

Estimations of pulmonary artery pressure, pulmonary vascular resistance and the effect of shunt on $Pao_2$ may be of use. The invasive nature, the risks involved and the difficulty in interpretation of these measurements means that they should not be used routinely but be reserved for specific indications in highly selected patients.

*Cardiac function tests*

The electrocardiogram (ECG) is simple, noninvasive and relatively cheap to perform. ECG stress test responses may provide more valuable information than a resting ECG in patients with coronary artery disease but it is more difficult to perform and it does not provide direct information on myocardial function. Further investigations with angiography, echocardiography or isotope studies should be carried out when specifically indicated, but again the invasive nature and risks determine that they should not become routine.

**Tests for day care patients**

Patients undergoing day care surgery expect the same high standard of care as any other patient, but the practical problems involved in obtaining results mean that tests are confined to the absolute minimum that are specifically indicated. Because of the physical status of most patients undergoing day care procedures there are few indications for X-rays and other investigations, but if patients who are more ill are treated, for example ASA III or IV, arrangements must be made for investigations to be performed well in advance.

# References

Asiddao, C. B., Donegan, J. H., Whitesell, R. C. and Kalbfleisch, J. H. (1982) Factors associated with perioperative complications during carotid endarterectomy. *Anesthesia and Analgesia*, **61**, 631–637

Association of Anaesthetists (1990) *Anaphylactic Reactions Associated with Anaesthesia*, Association of Anaesthetists, London

Bedford, R. F. and Feinstein, B. (1980) Hospital admission blood pressure: a predictor for hypertension following endotracheal intubation. *Anesthesia and Analgesia*, **59**, 367–370

Blogg, C. E. (1986) Halothane and the liver: the problem revisited and made obsolete. *British Medical Journal*, **1**, 1691–1692

Bradwell, A. R., Carmalt, M. H. B. and Whitehead, T. P. (1974) Explaining the unexpected abnormal results of biochemical investigations. *Lancet*, 2, 1071–1074

Brown, B. R. (1985) Halothane hepatitis revisited. *New England Journal of Medicine*, **313**, 1347–1348

Campbell, I. T. and Gosling, P. (1988) Preoperative biochemical screening: routine urine testing is good enough in patient under 50. *British Medical Journal*, 2, 803–804

Cohen, M. M. and Duncan, P. G. (1988) Physical status score and trends in anesthetic complications. *Journal of Clinical Epidemiology*, **41**, 83–90

Cormack, R. S. and Lehane, J. (1984) Difficult tracheal intubation in obstetrics. *Anaesthesia*, **39**, 1105–1111

Davies, S. C. and Brozovic, M. (1989) The presentation, management and prophylaxis of sickle cell disease. *Blood Reviews*, **3**, 29–44

Dresner, M. and Soni, N. (1989) Preoperative assessment. *Current Opinions in Anaesthesiology*, **2**, 701–708

Driksen, A. and Thomas, D. A. (1988) Cardiac predictors of death after noncardiac surgery evaluated by intention to treat. *British Medical Journal*, **297**, 1011–1013

Ellis, F. R. (1990) Predicting malignant hyperthermia. *British Journal of Anaesthesia*, **64**, 411–412

Fisher, A., Waterhouse, T. D. and Adams, A. P. (1975) Obesity: its relation to anaesthesia. *Anaesthesia*, **30**, 633–647

Fowkes, F. G. R., Davies, E. R., Evans, K. T., Green, G., Hartley, G., Hugh, A. E., Nolan, D. J., Power, A. L., Roberts, C. J. and Roylance, J. (1986) Multicentre trial of four strategies to reduce use of a radiological test. *Lancet*, **1**, 367–370

Fox, G. S., Whalley, D. G. and Bevan, D. R. (1981) Anaesthesia for the morbidly obese. Experience with 110 patients. *British Journal of Anaesthesia*, **53**, 811–815

Goldberger, A. L. and O'Konski, M. (1986) Utility of the routine electrocardiogram before surgery and on general hospital admission. *Annals of Internal Medicine*, **105**, 552–557

Goldman, L., Caldera, D. L., Nussbaum, S. R., Southwick, F. S., Krogstad, D., Murray, B. *et al.* (1977) Multifactorial index of cardiac risk in noncardiac surgical procedures. *New England Journal of Medicine*, **297**, 845–850

Gronert, G. A. (1980) Malignant hyperthermia. *Anesthesiology*, **53**, 395–423

Hackl, W., Mauritz, W., Schemper, M., Winkler, M., Sporn, P. and Steinbereithner, K. (1990) Prediction of malignant hyperthermia susceptibility: statistical evaluation of clinical signs. *British Journal of Anaesthesia*, **64**, 425–429

Hirsch, I. B., McGill, J. B., Cryer, P. E. and White, P. F. (1991) Perioperative management of surgical patients with diabetes mellitus. *Anesthesiology*, **74**, 346–359

Homi, J., Reynolds, J., Skinner, A., Hanna, W. and Sergant, G. (1979) General anaesthesia in sickle cell disease. *British Medical Journal*, **1**, 1599

Hudson, J. C., Dawson, K. S., Kane, F. R., Tyler, B. L. and Keenan, R. L. (1990) Are intraoperative complication rates influenced by ASA physical status, age, and emergency vs elective status? *Anesthesia and Analgesia*, **70**, S166

Kenna, J. G., Neuberger, J., Mieli-Vergani, G., Mowat, A. P. and Williams, R. (1987) Halothane hepatitis in children. *British Medical Journal*, **1**, 1209–1211

Lawrence, V. A. and Kroenke, K. (1988) The unproven utility of preoperative urinalysis – clinical use. *Archives of Internal Medicine*, **148**, 1370–1373

Lawrence, V. A., Page, C. P. and Harris, G. D. (1989) Preoperative spirometry before abdominal operations. A critical appraisal of its predictive value. *Archives of Internal Medicine*, **149**, 280–283

Lewin, I., Lerner, A. G., Green, S. H., Del Guercia, L. R. M. and Siegel, J. H. (1971) Physical class and physiologic status in the prediction of operative mortality in the aged sick. *Annals of Surgery*, **174**, 217–231

Mallampati, R. S., Gatt, S. P., Guginao, L. D., Desai, S. P., Waraksa, B., Freiberger, D. and Liu, P. L. (1985) A clinical sign to predict difficult tracheal intubation: a prospective study. *Canadian Anaesthetists' Society Journal*, **32**, 429–434

Marks, V. (1983) Clinical biochemistry nearer the patient. *British Medical Journal*, **286**, 1166–1167

McCleane, G. J. (1988) Urea and electrolyte measurement in preoperative surgical patients. *Anaesthesia*, **43**, 413–415

McKee, R. F. and Scott, E. M. (1987) The value of routine preoperative investigations. *Annals of the Royal College of Surgeons of England*, **69**, 160–162

Noble, D. W. and Yap, P. L. (1989) Editorial: Screening for antibodies to anaesthetics. No case for doing it yet. *British Medical Journal*, **2**, 2–3

Nunn, J. F., Melledge, J. S., Chen, D. and Dore, C. (1988) Respiratory criteria of fitness for surgery and anaesthesia. *Anaesthesia*, **43**, 543–551

Rabkin, S. W. and Horne, J. M. (1983) Preoperative electrocardiography: Effect of new abnormalities on clinical decisions. *Canadian Medical Association Journal*, **128**, 146–147

Rao, T. L. K., Jacobs, K. H. and El-Etr, A. A. (1983) Reinfarction following anesthesia in patients with myocardial infarction. *Anesthesiology*, **58**, 499–505

Robbins, J. A. and Mushlin, A. I. (1979) Preoperative evaluation of the healthy patient. *Medical Clinics of North America*, **63**, 1145–1156

Rohrer, M. J. Michelotti, M. C. and Nahrwold, D. L. (1988) A prospective evaluation of the efficacy of preoperative coagulation testing. *Annals of Surgery*, **208**, 554–557

Roizen, M. F. (1986) Routine preoperative evaluation. In *Anesthesia*, 2nd edn (ed. R. D. Miller), Churchill Livingstone, New York, p. 226

Royal College Working Party on the Effective Use of Diagnostic Radiology (1979) Preoperative chest radiology. National study by the Royal College of Radiologists. *Lancet*, **2**, 83–86

Samsoon, G. L. T. and Young, J. R. B. (1987) Difficult tracheal intubation: a retrospective study. *Anaesthesia*, **42**, 487–490

Sears, D. A. (1978) The morbidity of sickle cell trait: review of the literature. *American Journal of Medicine*, **64**, 1021–1036

Shaw, I. H. and Evans, J. M. (1988) Hospital anaesthesia and general practice. *British Medical Journal*, **2**, 1461–1464

Slogoff, S. and Keats, A. S. (1985) Does perioperative myocardial ischemia lead to postoperative myocardial infarction? *Anesthesiology*, **62**, 107–114

Tape, T. G. and Mushlin, A. I. (1986) The utility of routine chest radiographs. *Annals of Internal Medicine*, **104**, 663–670

Vacanti, C. J., Van Houten, R. J. and Hill, R. C. (1970) A statistical analysis of the relationship of physical status to postoperative mortality in 63,388 cases. *Anesthesia and Analgesia*, **49**, 564–566

Verma, P. K., Dhond, G. and Lawler, P. G. (1990) The interpretation of results by doctor technicians. *Anaesthesia*, **45**, 412

Walton, G. M. (1988) The cost benefit of routine pre-operative Hb investigations for oral surgery. *British Dental Journal*, **165**, 406–407

Wark, H. J. (1983) Post-operative jaundice in children. The influence of halothane. *Anaesthesia*, **38**, 237–242

Watkins, J. (1989) Second report from an anaesthetic reactions advisory service. *Anaesthesia*, **44**, 157–159

Weiss, M. E., Adkinson, N. F. and Hirshman, C. A. (1989) Evaluation of allergic drug reactions in the perioperative period. *Anesthesiology*, **71**, 483–486

White, A. and Kandor, P. L. (1975) Anatomical factors in difficult direct laryngoscopy. *British Journal of Anaesthesia*, **47**, 468–473

Wood, P. R. and Soni, N. (1989) Anaesthesia and substance abuse. *Anaesthesia*, **44**, 672–680

# 3

# Preoperative considerations

## Preoperative preparation

### Preparing for admission

Advice and information may have been given to the patient at the surgical clinic or at an anaesthetic assessment appointment. Advice will include alterations in pre-existing treatment, for example stopping aspirin therapy before major surgery because of the effect on haemostasis, or the correction of bleeding time by attention to anticoagulant management. Preoperative preparation may include intervention, such as dental treatment of carious, infected teeth before cardiac surgery. Changes in life style involving the consumption of tobacco and alcohol, or reduction in weight are sometimes desirable and in these situations patients only benefit from compliance with advice given weeks or even months before an operation. The following examples are of circumstances which may affect the outcome after anaesthesia and where benefit is sometimes achievable from action taken some time before the operation.

### Smoking

Smoking is a known cause of cardiac and respiratory disease, and is of special interest to the anaesthetist as both are associated with an increased perioperative risk.

The effect of nicotine is to raise heart rate, blood pressure and peripheral vascular resistance. This increases myocardial oxygen demand. Carbon monoxide, which is inhaled with the smoke, binds tightly to haemoglobin, forming carboxyhaemoglobin. Up to 15% of haemoglobin can be altered in this way, considerably decreasing available oxygen to the tissues. The respiratory effects of smoking are added to those already caused by a general anaesthetic resulting in an increased incidence of postoperative pulmonary complications. Long-term smoking can also depress immunological responses, and decrease the ability of the respiratory tract to clear secretions.

Benefits from stopping smoking can be obtained within 12 hours by a reduction in carboxyhaemoglobin levels. Six weeks or longer are needed for a substantial improvement in immune function, tracheo-bronchial clearance and reversible airways disease (Stein and Cassara, 1970; Jones, Rosen and Seymour, 1987).

Advice given in hospital may persuade patients to abstain from smoking permanently. About one-third of adult patients who present for surgery are cigarette smokers, and as a high proportion of surgically correctable disease is smoking-related, those patients who do permanently abstain will be much less at risk than those who continue to smoke. Thus this advice can have a preventative function for future health.

Pulse oximetry may not be a reliable monitor of oxygen saturation in heavy smokers as it can only distinguish two forms of haemoglobin, oxyhaemoglobin and reduced haemoglobin (Tremper and Barker, 1989). Carboxyhaemoglobin is interpreted as though almost all of it was oxyhaemoglobin. In the presence of carboxyhaemoglobin the pulse oximeter may therefore considerably overestimate oxygen saturation.

## Obesity

Obese patients have an increased immediate surgical morbidity and mortality (see Chapter 2), and the long-term outcome of the surgical procedure may also be affected. This is important in joint replacement, especially involving weight-bearing joints. If weight loss can be achieved in a controlled manner then benefits are to be expected. Significant weight reduction takes a long time to achieve, but where obesity directly affects outcome it may be used to indicate patient motivation when made a condition of surgery.

## Oral contraception

Studies performed in the 1970s show that women taking an oral contraceptive have a four- to sixfold increase in their relative risk of spontaneous venous thrombosis. The incidence of 0.2% in those taking the pill is none the less small and likely to be considerably smaller with the lower oestrogen pills now commonly prescribed. The incidence of deep vein thrombosis (DVT) after surgery in women taking the oral contraceptive and who did not receive prophylaxis has been reported to be between 1% and 20%. This should be compared with the 25% incidence for patients undergoing general surgery without prophylaxis to prevent a DVT and the 8% incidence in those who do receive prophylaxis (Sue-Ling and Hughes, 1988). The relatively low incidence of DVT in women on the pill is probably because they have few of the other risk factors. If the pill is stopped before surgery the young women may face an increased risk of becoming pregnant. Opinion is not uniform on policy towards women on the oral contraceptive and advice ranges from those who would like oestrogen-containing contraceptives to be discontinued four weeks before major elective surgery and subcutaneous low dose heparin prophylaxis considered when discontinuation is not possible (Guillebaud, 1985), to those who do not feel the pill should be stopped and that the routine use of prophylaxis is unnecessary (Sue-Ling and Hughes, 1988). It should be noted that manufacturers generally advise stopping the oral contraceptive for 6 weeks before an operation.

There are no data on the risk of postoperative venous thromboembolism in women on hormone replacement therapy (HRT); theoretically, however, there are unlikely to be increased risks (Whitehead and Whitehead, 1991). It should be noted that some manufacturers advise discontinuing HRT before surgery.

The following recommendations based on available information are for guidance and may need to be modified as further data becomes available.

1. Do not discontinue the pill prior to minor surgery of short duration and where early mobilization is possible, or when the pill does not contain oestrogen. Heparin prophylaxis is not indicated.
2. Consider discontinuing oestrogen-containing contraceptives 4 weeks before major elective surgery and in patients with additional risk factors. The oral contraceptive should be restarted at the first menses occurring at least 2 weeks after the procedure.
3. In patients before major surgery or who have additional risk factors and are still on the pill, prophylactic low dose subcutaneous heparin or other measures should be instituted.

*Exercise*

In normal subjects a programme of exercise increases maximum oxygen uptake and also the time for which exercise can be sustained. This is also true for patients with ischaemic heart disease and chronic heart failure (Coats et al., 1990). Exercise is also an important part of weight control, and has psychological benefits. Low physical fitness appears to be an important risk factor, both in men and women, for cardiovascular disease and cancer (Blair et al., 1989). Early mobilization, determination and self-motivation are all important for postoperative rehabilitation and a habit of regular exercise is almost certainly beneficial to those undergoing surgery and anaesthesia.

## Alcoholism

Alcohol has many side effects and some may increase the risk to patients during surgery and anaesthesia. These side effects include a diminished adrenocortical response to stress, impaired host defence mechanisms and bone marrow depression. Electrolyte and fluid imbalance can occur, as well as alterations in glucose metabolism. Chronic gastrointestinal upset is common, and liver disease, cardiomyopathy, alterations in the metabolism of anaesthetic and other drugs, and the alcohol withdrawal syndrome are other potential problems (Edwards, 1985).

Preoperative preparation for the confirmed alcoholic includes ensuring adequate nutrition and administering vitamin supplements, particularly thiamine, pyridoxine, nicotinic and pantothenic acids, and vitamin K. In the postoperative period symptoms of alcohol withdrawal will often start within 8 hours of abstention and must be anticipated in patients at risk.

## Upper respiratory tract infection

Upper respiratory tract infections (URTI) account in the United Kingdom for more than 50% of time lost from work through acute illness. Symptoms of URTI are often present in children during the winter months, and if always considered to be an indication for cancelling an operation this would result in many fewer children being subjected to anaesthesia. A child with an URTI given a general anaesthetic is four to seven times more likely than a child without this problem to have an adverse respiratory event in the perioperative period, and the chances of suffering such an event are increased if the child is intubated (Cohen and Cameron, 1991). The evidence is conflicting, however, as not all studies show an increased incidence of respiratory complications after minor procedures in children with uncomplicated URTI (Fennelly and Hall, 1990). Confusion also exists because the symptoms of a cold may herald the start of a more serious illness such as measles or pneumonia.

Recommendations have been published for the management of a child with an asymptomatic or mild URTI presenting for surgery (Cohen and Cameron, 1991). They are that elective procedures should be postponed for children under 1 year of age, and the risk/benefit of the surgical procedure should be considered on an individual basis for older children. Potential airway problems are less likely if intubation is not performed and in children older than 5 years of age. If the child is alert, physically active, apyrexial and has a clear chest to percussion and auscultation, then delay to minor surgery in children older than 1 year is probably not indicated. A more cautious approach is warranted with surgery that is major and where endotracheal intubation is to be performed. In these circumstances surgery should be delayed until several weeks after the symptoms of the URTI have subsided.

At present there is little evidence that anaesthesia in otherwise healthy adults suffering from an URTI leads to further severe complications, and the same guidelines as for children are reasonable. Any respiratory tract infection can be debilitating to a patient with chronic respiratory disease or with another serious illness, and for this reason it is important to consider the patient as a whole when deciding on the impact of the URTI on the decision to proceed with an anaesthetic.

## Preparation for day care surgery

Patients arriving at the hospital on the day of surgery should have received a considerable amount of information beforehand, either from the hospital or their general practitioner. This information is essential for the safe conduct of anaesthesia, and at the same time the hospital should be aware of any medical or other problem the patient has. In particular specific instructions on food and fluid intake should have been given and, more importantly, adhered to. Verbal instructions are liable to be forgotten or misinterpreted, and written instructions should also have been provided (Malins, 1978). Although this has been shown to improve compliance, there is no doubt that some patients deliberately ignore this advice. It is a prerequisite that patients treated on a day care basis are escorted home by a responsible adult in suitable transport and, where necessary, receive continuing postoperative care at home. If this care is not available it should be arranged with the general practitioner or local services. Instructions to the patient after anaesthesia should include permitted activities, the time when return to work is feasible, and when drugs, including alcohol and pain killers, may be taken, and when it is safe to drive and work machinery.

## Preoperative information for inpatients

Patients are entitled to be fully informed about the events that will affect them during their stay in hospital. This includes the ward routine, which is usually explained by the nursing staff, as well as a discussion of the surgical and anaesthetic proposals by the medical staff. The timetable of events is important, and should include the anticipated length of stay in hospital and the prospects for returning to normal activities.

### Surgery

The patient should understand the investigation or surgery contemplated, including the site and size of any incision. Discussion should cover the side effects, risks and possible long-term disabilities that may arise and should also include consideration of the available alternatives. The patient needs to have an idea of the duration of hospital stay and the likely time scale of rehabilitation and return to normal activity.

## Anaesthesia

All patients should have the opportunity to have the anaesthetic explained to them by someone who is familiar with the techniques, alternatives and side effects. The anaesthetic technique will be dictated by several considerations. These are primarily the particular procedure for which an anaesthetic is required and the medical condition of the patient. Other secondary, but none the less important, factors are the preference of the patient, the anaesthetist and the surgeon. The preferences of the doctors will take account of the experience and skill available to perform the procedures, and the availability of appropriate equipment, monitoring, assistance and recovery facilities. The choice between a regional or a general anaesthetic technique often illustrates this decision-making process.

## The consent form

Obtaining consent is merely confirmation that the information outlined above has been given and received. Thus it is not sufficient simply to get a consent form signed by a junior doctor. Informed consent can only be obtained if the patient has relevant information and understands the proposed procedure. The consent can be explicit or implied, verbal or written; a written consent form is helpful in providing documentary evidence. Unless a separate consent to anaesthesia is obtained then there is no record that anaesthetic considerations have been discussed. Recent suggestions on the format and aims of the consent form have been published in the United Kingdom in *A guide to consent for examination or treatment* (NHS Management Executive, 1990). Of interest to the anaesthetist is the statement that written consent should be obtained for anaesthesia and that the model consent form incorporates a section outlining the agreement by the patient to the type of anaesthesia – general, regional or sedation – that has been proposed.

## Informed consent

It is essential to obtain *informed* patient consent before any surgery or anaesthesia. One explanation of the ethical basis for this includes the desire to maximize good and minimize harm to the patient, the recognition of the individual's right to self-determination, the utilitarian goal of maximizing the good to society and lastly, and of secondary importance, the interests of the physician.

It has been stated that 'If a patient is fit to receive information and wishes to receive it, the doctor must "brief" the patient so that he can make a free and informed choice' (Scarman, 1986). It is not necessary to discuss fully all possible side effects and complications, but clinical judgement must be exercised in order to provide sufficient information to enable the patient to make a rational choice without raising unrealistic fears and concerns. In cases of genuine emergency medical care should take precedence over legal considerations, but only to the extent that those treatments necessary for the patient's immediate wellbeing are undertaken. In England any person of sound mind who has attained the age of 16 years may give a legally valid consent to surgery and anaesthesia. It is not clear whether a person who is younger than 16 years of age may also give consent. Many patients do not wish to know the full details of a procedure because it increases their fear of anaesthesia and surgery, or because they are truly not interested, while some patients require a full explanation and discussion. Others prefer to abrogate responsibility totally and leave the decision-making entirely to the doctors. In this latter circumstance we believe it is still the duty of the anaesthetist to offer some information. This should cover the nature of the anaesthetic and the side effects, as well as the potential risks and benefits of the techniques used. For example, if an epidural is used with a general anaesthetic and placed after induction then we feel the patient should at least be told that this is proposed, that a headache may occasionally ensue, and that waking up with temporarily paralysed legs is to be expected. Normally a fuller discussion of the indications, advantages and potential problems will be required. Similarly, if invasive monitoring is indicated, even if routinely used, such as with cardiac surgery, patients should be told that lines – central, arterial or pulmonary arterial – are going to be placed. It is also wise to mention the urinary catheter, gastrointestinal tube, drainage tubes and the like, and to indicate the form of dressing that will be applied.

Sometimes the patient will want to know more about the anaesthetic. In the examples above questions may be asked about the complications of epidural anaesthesia or the hazards of inserting a central line. Arrangements should exist to answer such questions, and to address fears and worries that the patient may have. The best person to do this is the anaesthetist who will be giving the anaesthetic. If this cannot be arranged, then another anaesthetist should be available.

This pre-anaesthetic discussion should take place well before the time of surgery and, at the latest, before administration of the premedication. If there are specific aspects relevant to the anaesthetic that are peculiar to a particular patient then it is prudent that this is recorded. The record could include the preoperative assessment, any decisions or action taken, such as extra monitoring or reserving an intensive care bed, and the fact that the patient was aware of potential problems. It should also include the name of the interviewer and the date and time at which the interview took place. If epidural anaesthesia is planned it has been suggested that anaesthetists should explain wherever possible the limitations of the procedure and discuss the potential complications. Good effective communication will help prevent misunderstandings that could lead to litigation. If action against an anaesthetist is taken then a successful defence depends heavily on accurate contemporaneous records (Palmer, 1988). When the patient, because of his or her medical condition, is at a substantially increased risk from an anaesthetic for a given procedure, it is wise to note this. In these circumstances it is obviously false to pretend to a patient that a risk does not exist, and we believe that patients are entitled to a straightforward and accurate account of the situation.

## Psychological preparations

There is a further important benefit to the patient of a full discussion and explanation of the procedures to be undergone. Evidence suggests that anxiety is allayed as effectively by a preoperative visit as by medication, and furthermore, in some cases recovery may be quicker, less postoperative analgesia is required and patients leave hospital earlier (Egbert *et al.*, 1963, 1964; Leigh, Walker and Janaganathan, 1977; Anderson, 1987). A tape containing 'therapeutic suggestions' of encouragement and positive outcome played to patients under a general anaesthetic also apparently aids recovery and decreases hospital stay (Evans and Richardson, 1988) and decreases morphine requirements in the early postoperative period (McLintock *et al.*, 1990). Preoperative anxiety primarily appears to reflect the patient's personality and method of coping with problems (Domar, Everett and Keller, 1989). The anxieties commonly focus on the period before transfer to the operating theatre, the possibility of intraoperative awareness, not recovering from the anaesthetic, and postoperative pain and nausea (McCleane and Cooper, 1990). These topics can be discussed with the patient at the preoperative visit.

## Rejection of medical advice

There are occasions when an adult will decide to act against medical advice and refuse appropriate treatment – when a Jehovah's Witness refuses to have a blood transfusion, for example (Benson, 1989). The wishes of an adult who is of sound mind should always be respected. In this circumstance it is vital that the patient's request is written into the notes and is independently witnessed, and in many hospitals special forms exist to cover this situation.

The position for the children of Jehovah's Witnesses is less clear. It is a criminal offence in England for anyone over 16 who has custody, charge or care of a child under 16 wilfully to expose that child to ill treatment or neglect or to expose him or her to unnecessary suffering or injury to health. Where the patient is a minor and the parent or guardian refuses permission for life-saving therapy, decisions ultimately need to be taken on the basis that it is the child and not the parent who is the patient. It is possible to get the patient taken into care, but in the absence of such an order and when time is short, the life-saving therapy should be instituted without delay. The principle is that until and unless the patient can make decisions for himself or herself, then no one should overrule the right to administer treatment in circumstances where otherwise the patient who is suffering from a remediable state would die or be at risk of suffering permanent harm. As well as minors, this principle applies to the mentally handicapped, the seriously injured or when no parent or guardian is available for a child.

## Food and fluid restrictions

### General anaesthesia

The purpose of restricting oral intake is an attempt to ensure that the stomach is empty in order to minimize the risk of a patient aspirating stomach contents and to reduce the danger of postoperative vomiting. The fact that aspiration still remains a major cause of anaesthetic-related morbidity and mortality attests to the importance of such measures as well as the fact that they are not totally effective. In starved patients undergoing elective surgery it is not uncommon to find residual gastric volumes of more than 25 ml at a pH of less than 2.5 (Ong, Pahlnuik and Cumming, 1978). There are some circumstances when gastric emptying is impaired, and these are listed in Table 3.1. When any of these factors are present patients should be assumed to have full stomachs (Bricker, McLuckie and Nightingale, 1989) and precautions taken to minimize the danger by therapy to decrease gastric volume and acidity, as well as the use of a rapid induction sequence for general anaesthesia or selected local or regional techniques.

**Table 3.1   Factors slowing gastric emptying**

| | | |
|---|---|---|
| Pain | Anxiety | Obesity |
| Pregnancy | Alcohol | Trauma |
| Analgesics | Diabetes | Myxoedema |
| Peptic ulceration | | Electrolyte disturbances |

The stomach is an organ with a daily secretion of about 2000 ml and it is wrong to assume that it will remain empty just because nothing is put into it. Gastric emptying times will be affected by an ingested meal, being more prolonged for solids and hyper- or hypo-osmolar liquids. It is important to avoid the presence of solids in the stomach and food should therefore not be given in the 4 hours, and probably in the 6 hours before an elective procedure. Remember that if there are factors that delay gastric motility the stomach may not be empty, no matter how long the period of starvation (Table 3.1). Traditional teaching has been to restrict fluid for at least 4–6 hours before surgery. A healthy adult will empty his or her stomach of liquids with a half time of 10–20 minutes. Several recent studies have indicated that drinking clear fluids about 2 hours before the operation decreases gastric volume by promoting gastric emptying and may increase pH by diluting gastric juices (Maltby *et al.*, 1986, Sutherland *et al.*, 1987, Agarwal, Chari and Singh, 1989). In otherwise normal adults, fluid up to 2 hours before an elective operation is therefore not contraindicated and may in fact be beneficial. Similar findings apply to children and adolescents (Cote, 1990; Miller, 1990; Splinter, Stewart and Muir, 1990) and by extension we would suggest that in infants and children food and milk is withheld within 4 hours of an anaesthetic but that clear fluids may be continued up to within 2 hours of the procedure. Predicting the time of the start of an operation is an uncertain art which becomes more difficult as the operating list progresses. It is essential that the minimum times from fluid ingestion to induction are not violated. It should be noted that many pre-anaesthetic medications affect gastric emptying and further research is needed in this area.

## Local or regional anaesthesia

The same precautions that are applied to patients before a general anaesthetic should be used where there is any risk that protective reflexes may be depressed for other reasons. This applies to all patients given sedative or potent analgesic drugs, where large doses of local anaesthetic are to be used, or where a regional or local block may directly affect the protective reflexes. In practice this means all patients receiving a major regional block, such as an epidural or spinal, or local blocks to the airway, larynx or pharynx. It may be safe practice to apply the same considerations when performing intravenous regional anaesthesia (IVRA, Biers block) and during infiltration anaesthesia for anything other than the most minor of lesions.

## Adverse effects of fluid restriction

Prolonged fluid restriction will cause dehydration. This will be compounded in patients who are already dehydrated. Examples of this are those who have preoperative bowel washouts, those on chronic diuretic therapy, and those in a poor nutritional state. In addition, patients with urinary frequency or incontinence often voluntarily restrict their fluid intake. In these patients insertion of an intravenous cannula may be more difficult, and hypotension at induction is probably more common than in other patients. There is evidence to suggest that patients who are fluid-deprived recover less well after a general anaesthetic and may suffer more commonly from minor complications such as headache. All these disadvantages can be avoided by the use of preoperative intravenous fluid therapy or by decreasing the length of time patients are fluid-restricted before the operation.

Prolonged restriction of oral intake may also result in hypoglycaemia. Most adults compensate well but this may be a problem in children (Miller, 1990), thus it is wise to include dextrose in the infusion fluid of small children.

## Prophylaxis to prevent complications

Measures can be taken in the preoperative period or during the anaesthetic itself to prevent or minimize some potential complications of anaesthesia and surgery. Some of the conditions where prophylaxis is of benefit are considered below.

### Deep vein thrombosis (DVT)

A DVT may cause postoperative discomfort and long-term sequelae but is not of itself life-threatening. The real danger of a DVT is that a pulmonary embolus may result (Bell and Simon, 1982). Studies have shown embolization in up to 60% of cases of DVT, but the true incidence of embolization is probably nearer 15–20% (Bell and Simon, 1982). Without prophylaxis fatal postoperative emboli occur in 0.1–0.8% of patients undergoing elective general surgery (Goucke, 1989). The clinical diagnosis of pulmonary emboli is difficult and they almost certainly contribute to more postoperative deaths than is generally recorded (Sandler and Martin, 1989), thus making them one of the most important causes of avoidable postoperative mortality. The problem was highlighted by the report of the Confidential Enquiry into Perioperative Deaths (CEPOD) (Buck, Devlin and Lunn, 1987) where the need to provide adequate prophylaxis was discussed. Table 3.2 outlines the associated risk factors.

Methods of DVT prevention are detailed in Table 3.3 (Goucke, 1989; Dehring and Arens, 1990). It is the responsibility of the anaesthetist to consult with the surgical team to ensure that adequate prophylaxis is administered. For most procedures the combination of early ambulation, graduated compression stockings and low-dose

Table 3.2    Risk factors associated with pulmonary emboli (PE)

Age – more common in adults than children
    – more common older than 50 years
Cardiac disease – AF, congestive failure, rheumatic, arteriosclerotic, bacterial,
    hypertensive
Obesity
Pregnancy and the puerperium
Oral contraceptives
Smoking
Metabolic disease – diabetes, homocystinuria, Behçet's syndrome
History of previous DVT or PE
Immobilization and pressure on calves
Trauma – especially to hip and pelvis, major burns
Surgery – especially gynaecological, major orthopaedic, abdominal
Neoplasms

subcutaneous heparin will be sufficient. Dextran has been shown to be effective as prophylaxis particularly during hip surgery. Regional anaesthesia will decrease the frequency of DVT during hip surgery and this should be considered by the anaesthetist when selecting a technique.

Table 3.3    Prevention of deep vein thrombosis (DVT)

Early postoperative ambulation
Leg elevation
Graduated compression (TED) stockings
Active and passive leg exercise
Limb pneumatic compression
Electrical calf muscle stimulation
Warfarin anticoagulant prophylaxis
Low-dose heparin 5000 i.u. subcutaneously 12 hourly
Dextran 70
Regional anaesthesia

## Aspiration of gastric contents

Aspiration of gastric contents accounts for up to 20% of anaesthetic-related major morbidity and death and the mortality after a significant aspiration remains high. In addition to those obviously at risk, such as from intestinal obstruction, the chances of an aspiration are increased in all cases where oral food or fluids have recently been taken, where gastric emptying is slowed (see Table 3.1), where patients' reflexes are obtunded or where gastro-oesophageal reflux exists. Although emphasis is quite rightly placed on the increased risk to pregnant women, it should be remembered that even in a patient prepared for elective surgery considerable quantities of stomach contents may be present and silent regurgitation can occur in up to 25% of these patients (Miller and Anderson, 1988). Prophylaxis should be given routinely before anaesthesia, both general and regional, to pregnant women during the second and third trimester of pregnancy and up until 2 weeks after delivery. Although it has been suggested that this should be extended to all patients receiving a general anaesthetic (Coombs, 1983), this has not received general support (Editorial, 1989b) and most anaesthetists will restrict treatment to those patients with added risk factors.

Although emphasis is placed on the risk at induction of anaesthesia, the hazard remains in the immediate recovery period. Although a cuffed endotracheal tube with the cuff properly inflated provides good protection of the airway, soiling of the respiratory tract is still possible. In patients with obtunded reflexes or a diminished level of consciousness such as those suffering from a drug overdose, a head injury or a cerebrovascular accident, the risk is ever present. The aim of prophylaxis is threefold; to decrease the volume of gastric contents, to increase its pH and to promote gastric emptying. As a rule of thumb it is often quoted that an undesirable combination is when the volume of the gastric aspirate is greater than 25 ml and the pH is less than 2.5. Methods of prophylaxis are shown in Table 3.4 (Joyce, 1987). Cimetidine has a short duration of action and is associated with several undesirable side effects, including hypotension and alteration of the metabolism of other drugs, thus ranitidine is commonly preferred. Although anticholinergic drugs such as atropine and glycopyrrolate reduce acidity of stomach contents, they are not as effective as other methods and have the undesirable effect of lowering oesphageal sphincter pressure.

**Table 3.4    Prophylaxis against acid aspiration**

1. No oral intake (particularly solids) for 4–6 hr preoperatively

2. Antacids – 0.3 M sodium citrate, 30 ml 15–20 minutes before surgery

3. Histamine-2 (H2) blockers – decrease acid secretion
    Cimetidine 300 mg p.o. the night before + 300 mg p.o. 4 hr preop. or 300 mg i.m./i.v. 1 hr preop.
    Ranitidine 150 mg p.o. the night before + 150 mg p.o. 4 hr preop. or 50 mg i.m./i.v. 1 hr preop.

4. Metoclopramide – stimulates gastric emptying, increases oespohageal sphincter pressure, antiemetic
    10 mg p.o. 2 hr preop. or i.m./i.v. 1 hr preop.
A combination of these methods is commonly used

5. Protection of the airway
    Rapid sequence induction including cricoid pressure endotracheal intubation posture, on left side, head down

*Prophylaxis against infection*

Antibiotic prophylaxis has been shown to be effective in reducing the incidence of infection in many surgical procedures (Noone, 1988). The use of antimicrobial agents can have undesirable side effects, including allergic reactions, toxic side effects and the potential for superinfection with resistant organisms, and they are expensive drugs. Thus antimicrobial prophylaxis should not be considered a substitute for poor surgical technique, and its use should be restricted to circumstances where clear benefit has been demonstrated.

Indications for prophylaxis include operations where the surgical wound is sited in areas likely to be contaminated by gut, skin, or other organ microflora, or when an infection would cause catastrophic complications. It is important that adequate concentrations of the appropriate antibiotic are present in the tissues and blood at the time of bacterial soiling and for this reason antibiotics are usually given intravenously at induction, and continued for a period thereafter. The particular antimicrobials will depend on the likely contaminants.

**Table 3.5   Antibiotic prophylaxis of infective endocarditis**

---

1. Routine adult prophylaxis for procedures under anaesthesia
   AMOXYCILLIN: 3 g orally repeated post procedure or 1 g i.m. plus 0.5 g
                         orally/i.m. 6 hours later

If allergic to penicillin:
   ERYTHROMYCIN: 1.5 g orally, and 0.5 g 6 hours later
or
   CLINDAMYCIN: 600 mg orally

2. Adult prophylaxis in special circumstances
   (a) Gastrointestinal procedures
   (b) Genitourinary procedures
   (c) Patients at special risk (prosthetic valves or previous endocarditis)

   AMOXYCILLIN: 1 g i.m. plus 0.5 g orally/i.m. 6 hours later
plus
   GENTAMICIN: 120 mg i.m.

If allergic to penicillin:
   VANCOMYCIN: 1 g slow i.v. over 60 minutes
plus
   GENTAMICIN: 120 mg i.v.

---

Adapted from the Endocarditis Working Party of the British Society for Antimicrobial Chemotherapy (1990) *Lancet*, **i**, 88–89.
Doses for children should be given on a body weight basis. I.v. injections may be substituted for i.m.

Current recommendations for antibiotic prophylaxis specifically against infective endocarditis are detailed in Table 3.5. Patients who need to be protected are those with congenital or acquired structural abnormality of the heart, including hypertrophic cardiomyopathy, but patients with coronary artery disease, including those who have had coronary bypass surgery, are not at risk. The standard adult prophylaxis is amoxycillin (3 g oral, 1 g i.m.), with erythromycin or clindamycin as an alternative for patients who are allergic to penicillin. For genitourinary or gastrointestinal surgery, and with special risk patients with prosthetic heart valves or who have had previous endocarditis, gentamicin (120 mg) should be added, and vancomycin (1 g by slow infusion) should be substituted for amoxycillin in patients allergic to penicillin (Endocarditis Working Party ..., 1990). In most surgical patients it will be possible, and much kinder, to give the antibiotics by the intravenous rather than the intramuscular route.

## Adrenocortical suppression

It is feared that patients on steroid therapy, or who have recently stopped such treatment, will have their normal adrenocortical response to stress suppressed by the exogenous steroid given for treatment of various conditions. Although steroid therapy may undoubtedly have this effect, evidence demonstrating that this alters patient outcome is scarce. Several anaesthetic regimes, such as a high epidural block with local anaesthetic or large doses of opiate, will normally suppress the response and if side effects, such as hypotension, do occur it is difficult to show that a lack of steroid is the direct cause. Although there is relatively little risk in giving steroid prophylaxis to ensure adequate levels the undesirable side effects can include infection, decreased wound healing, hypertension, fluid retention and stress ulceration. There is probably no need to give replacement therapy if steroids were halted more than 2 months before surgery. In response to stress the body produces a maximum of about 300 mg of hydrocortisone per 24 hours, and there is no logic in giving more than this to manage adrenocortical suppression. A reasonable dosage regime is therefore 50 mg 4-hourly or 80 mg 6-hourly. If steroid therapy with dosage in excess of normal requirements continues into the postoperative period, then extra prophylaxis is unlikely to be necessary.

## Asthma and hyperallergy

Patients with a history of asthma or allergy are four to five times more likely than the normal population to have an 'anaphylactoid' response to drugs, including anaesthetic agents. However a history of allergy is not a reliable predictor, and most incidents of anaphylactoid response occur in people who do not have a positive history, and conversely the vast majority of people with such a history have uneventful anaesthesia. The only relevant valid factor that will predict whether a patient is likely to have an anaphylactoid reaction to a drug is a history of a previous reaction to that drug. If prophylaxis is considered necessary then pretreatment with $H_1$ and $H_2$ histamine receptor antagonists and steroids should be considered. Cromoglycate may be useful in preventing the pulmonary effects. In cases where there are major cardiovascular or respiratory manifestations of an anaphylactoid reaction, adrenaline is the most valuable drug for immediate resuscitation, and it must not be withheld.

*Respiratory complications: the role of preoperative chest physiotherapy*

The incidence of postoperative pulmonary complications varies from 6% to 80% and is particularly associated with upper abdominal and thoracic surgery, patients of advanced age and those with pre-existing lung disease. If physiotherapy is to be of value in preventing these complications it should be instituted prior to surgery, and continued thereafter into the postoperative period. There is no evidence that routine postural drainage, percussion and vibration is of value in younger patients with healthy lungs, even when undergoing upper abdominal surgery. In those patients with pre-existing pathology the evidence of the efficacy of physiotherapy alone is poor, although there appears to be some benefit when combined with bronchodilators in patients with chronic respiratory disease, or where copious sputum or acute atelectasis is present (Stein and Cassara, 1970; Selsby, 1990; Selsby and Jones, 1990). Other measures are often useful to improve chest pathology, and patients who smoke should abstain, ideally for several weeks or possibly months in order to gain maximum benefit, and appropriate antibiotic therapy may be indicated to control respiratory tract infection in patients with chronic bronchitis. Surprisingly physiotherapy is not without side effects, for it may cause bronchospasm and produce hypoxaemia.

*Minor postoperative morbidity*

The surgeon is often judged by the size of the surgical scar and the anaesthetist by the incidence of anaesthetic-related side effects. It is important and worthwhile to minimize the number and severity of these complications. The most troublesome anaesthetic-related complications are those likely to delay immediate recovery, and these are nausea and vomiting, pain, syncope, hypoventilation and drowsiness. The anaesthetic agents and technique used will affect the incidence of these side effects and this is considered further below. Other morbidity less likely to affect recovery, but none the less troublesome to the patient, can be related to the anaesthetic. Sore throats and suxamethonium-related myalgia are two such problems which are examined.

*Nausea and vomiting*   Vomiting is common after a general anaesthetic and is experienced by 20–40% of patients. Various factors affect the incidence, including sex, age, obesity, gastric dilatation, type of operation, anaesthetic drugs, duration of anaesthesia, postoperative medication and also pain, sudden movement or position change, hypotension and a previous history of motion sickness (Palazzo and Strunin, 1984a,b; Editorial, 1989a). Vomiting is rarely the result of a single factor and it is difficult to reduce the incidence substantially, especially in certain procedures such as strabismus surgery and operations on the middle ear. Many studies have been performed with limited success using selected anaesthetic techniques or prophylactic antiemetics in an attempt to decrease the incidence. Of the antiemetics, droperidol is probably the prophylactic agent of choice (Palazzo and Strunin, 1984b). An intravenous dose of 1.25 mg is effective in adults and causes few side effects. One technique that has been shown to work in some situations is stimulation of the P6 acupuncture point. This technique deserves further consideration if for no other reason than that it lacks toxic side effects (Dundee and Fee, 1989).

*Pain in recovery*   The anaesthetist should aim to provide the patient with adequate analgesia at the end of the operation without dangerous or unecessary sedation, or respiratory depression. Pain in the immediate postoperative period will partly depend on the amount of analgesia administered during a procedure and the potential for an operation to result in pain should be a consideration in deciding on drug dosage. The use of regional or local anaesthetic techniques is often an extremely effective means of providing postoperative analgesia without the systemic effects, such as sedation and nausea, that may accompany the use of potent analgesic drugs.

*Hypoventilation and drowsiness*   Hypoventilation and drowsiness are considered together as they both usually result from a relative overdose of anaesthetic drugs. Central nervous system depressants such as inhalational anaesthetic agents, opioids and benzodiazepines will all make patients sleepy and will depress respiration. Hypoventilation is also caused by inadequate recovery of muscle power after paralysis with a muscle relaxant. These side effects can be minimized by careful and skilled administration of anaesthesia complemented by anticipation of the likely course and duration of the operation.

*Syncope*   This side effect is often caused by the combination of a dehydrated patient and the residual effect of the anaesthetic; thus hypovolaemia is exacerbated by vasodilatation and impairment of cardiovascular reflexes resulting in a fall in cardiac output. The question of fluid therapy has already been considered. An intravenous infusion should be instituted if a patient is fluid-restricted for more than a few hours before an operation, if the procedure is likely to produce loss of fluid, or if the patient is unlikely to be able to drink within a short time of the end of the anaesthetic.

*Sore throat*    The causes of a postoperative sore throat are complicated and multifactorial. The quoted incidence ranges from 0% to 22% in nonintubated patients, and up to 100% in those who are intubated. When a tube is passed the incidence is related to the size and design of the tube and cuff, the materials of which the tube is constructed, cuff pressures and lubricants (Sprague and Archer, 1987; Alexander and Leach, 1989; Monroe, Gravenstein and Saga-Rumley, 1990). The lowest incidence of sore throat follows the use of a tube with a low cuff area in contact with the trachea and with a low cuff pressure. The laryngeal mask airway (Brain, 1983), somewhat surprisingly, results in a similar incidence of sore throat to a simple face mask. Contributory factors to be avoided include dry inspired gases and instrumentation and excessive suction to the pharynx. The use of throat packs or the presence of a nasogastric tube increases the incidence of sore throats.

*Suxamethonium-induced myalgia*    Approximately half the patients given suxamethonium experience postoperative muscle pains, although values as low as 5% and as high as 80% have been recorded (Pace, 1990). The pain in certain individuals can be severe and disabling, and those particularly likely to suffer are young, fit patients who are rapidly mobilized after surgery. Several pretreatments have been advocated in an attempt to decrease this incidence. None will completely prevent the pains but pretreatment with nondepolarizing muscle relaxants, diazepam, or lignocaine all reduce the incidence by about 30%. Pretreatment with suxamethonium (self-taming) does not appear to be effective.

   Because of the high incidence of morbidity associated with the use of suxamethonium, as a general rule the authors believe that it should be avoided unless specifically indicated, such as for situations when rapid intubation is necessary because of the risk of aspiration, or when endotracheal intubation is required for a procedure of short duration.

# The optimum time for surgery

A patient undergoing surgery and anaesthesia should be in the best possible physical condition before the anaesthetic begins. Although in practice this cannot mean the enforcement of unrealistic goals on unwilling patients, such as a severe diet on moderately obese patients or refusing to treat smokers unless they abstain, the preoperative assessment does provide an opportunity to point out the increased risks associated with these conditions. It is, however, obligatory to optimize the treatment of coexisting medical conditions, for example, heart failure, cardiac ischaemia, epilepsy, asthma and diabetes. Even when contemplating emergency surgery, time is often available and can be profitably spent preparing the patient. The most obvious and important treatment is instituting fluid and electrolyte replacement. In the very rare cases where surgery cannot be delayed at all, the induction of anaesthesia should begin so the operation can proceed while the anaesthetist continues the process of resuscitation at the same time. Good communication and cooperation between the surgeon and anaesthetist are essential in these circumstances.

If patients scheduled for routine surgery are postponed unnecessarily, not only will inconvenience, frustration and expense result, but physical and social harm may also follow. The physical harm will occur from the increased risk of deep vein thrombosis and pneumonia in patients confined to bed, and from the progression of their disease. Hospitalization, especially in elderly patients, can lead to dependence and disorientation. Thus scheduled operations should only be postponed in exceptional circumstances.

# Premedication

## *Preoperative medication*

The anaesthetist has many objectives when prescribing pre-anaesthetic medication (Table 3.6), only some of which may be desirable in a particular patient. The main aim must be to achieve an effect before the patient arrives in the anaesthetic room, although some of the objectives for which premedication is given may also be achieved by intravenous drug administration at induction or during the anaesthetic. Premedication should never be routine, and drug choice, route of administration and dose must be tailored to the individual patient, taking into account the patient's age, weight, physical status, degree of apprehension, previous experience with premedicants, allergies and preferences. It is also necessary to bear in mind the preferences and techniques of the anaesthetist, the procedure to be performed, and the anticipated time the patient will remain in hospital.

Anxiolysis is probably the commonest reason for administering preoperative medication. It should be remembered that a visit by the anaesthetist may be effective in allaying anxiety by providing information and explanation, and by allowing patients to express their fears and concerns. If premedication is thought necessary it may be useful to administer a sedative the night before the operation in order to help the patient sleep. On the day of operation premedication is

**Table 3.6    Aims of pre-anaesthetic medication**

1. Premedication for anaesthesia
   Allay anxiety
   Achieve sedation
   Induce some amnesia
   Provide analgesia
   Prevent nausea and vomiting
   Minimize secretions
   Reduce requirement for anaesthetic agents

2. Specific prophylaxis to prevent
   Aspiration – increase gastric pH, decrease gastric volumes, increase gastric emptying
   Anaphylactoid reactions
   Infection
   DVTs
   Side effects of adrenocortical suppression

3. To continue therapy for existing medical conditions, e.g. diabetes, epilepsy, asthma etc.

commonly given by the oral or intramuscular route. The route will depend on the medication chosen, the preferences of the patient and factors directly affecting the route of administration. As an example, oral premedication is inappropriate in a patient with an oesophageal stricture or poor gastric emptying, whereas an intramuscular injection is contraindicated in a patient with abnormal coagulation.

There are adverse effects to all premedicants and many patients will be content to forego all preoperative medication in exchange for a quicker recovery. In particular premedication should not be administered without specific indication to the elderly, the confused or those with central nervous system depression.

## Care of the premedicated patient

The pre-anaesthetic medication must be the last part of the preparation undergone by the patient before induction of anaesthesia. It is quite wrong to continue preparation in a premedicated patient, and in particular they should not be questioned, moved or made to sign documents except with the express permission of the anaesthetist. Any attempt to gain informed consent at this time would be invalid. After a patient has been given the preoperative medication observations must ensure that no harm ensues from the effects of the drugs, and that no adverse response has occurred. It is the duty of the anaesthetist to prescribe appropriate premedication for the individual patient so that vital protective reflexes are not depressed. The nurses have the responsibility of caring for the premedicated patient and must be aware of the effect of the medication. The commonest, and desired, effect will be drowsiness and amnesia, and for this reason patients must be confined to a bed or trolley. If heavy sedation is aimed at, which is common practice in patients about to undergo cardiac surgery, the premedication increases the likelihood of hypoxia and this can be minimized by giving oxygen via a face mask until the induction of anaesthesia.

Some anaesthetists prefer to give little or no premedication to sedate their patients. This is routine practice with many patients having minor surgery in day care units. These patients should sit or lie in a quiet and calm location until called for surgery.

## Premedication in children

The requirements of premedication are very different in young children. In the very young there will be no appreciation of future events and any anxiety displayed will be the result of the strange surroundings and unknown people, together with any effects of the illness for which the procedure is required. Many anaesthetists still prefer to administer an anticholinergic drug to neonates and small infants. This will dry secretions and thus protect the airway, and help prevent the bradycardia that commonly follows induction or the use of suxamethonium. Opiates and sedatives should not be given to neonates and must be used with care in small children, for there is a real risk that they may induce respiratory depression which could also last into the postoperative period.

Some anaesthetists administer barbiturates rectally as a premedicant/induction agent. The drug takes about 10 minutes to work and the time of the instillation of the drug should be treated as the time of induction of anaesthesia and therefore appropriate monitoring should be used and great care exercised during this period.

Older children must be treated as intelligent beings and need to be given a proper explanation of what is happening to them. Placation with platitudes or downright lies may permanently damage the psyche of a sensitive child. It should be remembered that children can also interpret words and actions in unexpected ways. For example the phrase 'I will put you to sleep' may be confused with the words used by the vet when putting down the old and infirm family pet, so the words must be carefully chosen and accompanied by sufficient explanation. It may be reassuring for the child to be told how they will go to sleep, that someone will be looking after them throughout the procedure, that they will not wake up or feel any pain during the operation, and that their parents or loved ones will be nearby when they awake.

# From ward to theatre

*Preoperative checklist*

Before the patient leaves the ward certain formalities should be carried out. A senior nurse should correctly identify the patient to the porter and escort by reference to a wrist band with name and hospital number which matches that on the hospital notes and consent form. The consent form must state the procedure to be performed and must be properly completed and be available in the records. The nature of the operation or procedure should be clearly indicated and if the procedure is unilateral the side of operation must be clearly stated on the consent form and ideally the site marked on the patient by the surgeons. Any preoperative medications must have been given and the drug chart checked and signed. All items of jewellery and prostheses, including dentures, contact lenses, false nails, hearing aids etc. must be removed and the patient should wear no make-up or nail polish. The ward supervision during the preceding hours should ensure that patients have not taken oral fluid or food for the specified period. Ideally a formal checklist is completed and signed to witness that the ward staff have completed their part of the preoperative preparation. None of this should entail disturbing the patient by unnecessary movement or by questioning, for the replies of a premedicated patient cannot be relied upon.

*Escort*

All patients should be taken from the ward to the operating theatres by a trained escort. There is often a period of waiting before anaesthesia starts and it is desirable for the patient to have an understanding and sympathetic companion who is also familiar with the working of the theatre, and one who is capable of recognizing and dealing with complications that may arise. There is a distinct advantage if the patient is escorted by a nurse from the ward for in this case the patient is accompanied by a familiar person, one who should be able to assist if there are questions relating to the preoperative ward management. It is usually beneficial for a parent to accompany a child to theatre, but if the parent is clearly upset or is unsettling the child, there should be no hesitation by the anaesthetist in asking the parent to leave.

There have been cases, fortunately rare, when a woman has been sexually abused under the influence of anaesthesia or heavy sedation. More commonly it is possible for a woman to imagine or dream that such an event has taken place. In order to protect both the patient and the doctor it is advisable that when a female patient is examined or given sedative or anaesthetic drugs that she is never left without a female companion. Sensitivity to the feelings of the patient is also necessary when intimate contact is required, such as when attaching chest ECG electrodes. This in no way reflects on the high professional standards of male nurses, but is merely a matter of common sense.

Patients for day care surgery who have not received any premedication can walk to the operating theatre and be assisted on to the operating table. Other patients are taken on an easily wheeled bed or trolley. Narrow trolleys should have sides to prevent patients falling out, and beds without sides should be restricted to patients who are not at risk of inadvertently moving. In all cases it is ideal if the patient is accompanied by two escorts, one at each end of the bed or trolley. With patients at risk of falling out of the trolley two escorts are mandatory. These patients include the young, the confused and the heavily sedated.

## Notes and X-rays

All relevant information should accompany the patient to the theatres. This includes notes, X-rays and drug charts. If these are not available in the theatres the operation should be delayed until they are found. The surgical ward is responsible for making sure these documents are with the patient.

# References

Agarwal, A., Chari, P. and Singh, H. (1989) Fluid deprivation before operation. The effect of a small drink. *Anaesthesia*, **44**, 632–634

Alexander, C. A. and Leach, A. B. (1989) Incidence of sore throats with the laryngeal mask. *Anaesthesia*, **44**, 791

Anderson, E. A. (1987) Preoperative preparation for cardiac surgery facilitates recovery, reduces psychological distress, and reduces the incidence of acute postoperative hypertension. *Journal of Consulting and Clinical Psychology*, **55**, 513–520

Bell, W. R. and Simon, T. L. (1982) Current status of pulmonary thromboembolic disease: pathophysiology, diagnosis, prevention, and treatment. *American Heart Journal*, **103**, 239–261

Benson, K. T. (1989) The Jehovah's Witness patient: considerations for the anesthesiologist. *Anesthesia and Analgesia*, **69**, 647–656

Blair, S. N., Kohl, H. W., Paffenbarger, R. S. Jr, Clark, D. G., Cooper, K. H. and Gibbons, L. W. (1989) Physical fitness and all-cause mortality. A prospective study of healthy men and women. *Journal of the American Medical Association*, **262**, 2395–2401

Brain, A. I. (1983) The laryngeal mask – a new concept in airway management. *British Journal of Anaesthesia*, **55**, 801–805

Bricker, S. R. W., McLuckie, A. and Nightingale, D. A. (1989) Gastric aspirates after trauma in children. *Anaesthesia*, **44**, 721–724

Buck, N., Devlin, H. B. and Lunn, J. N. (1987) *Report of the Confidential Enquiry into Perioperative Deaths*, Nuffield Provincial Hospitals Trust/King's Fund, London

Preoperative considerations 69

Coats, A. J. S., Adampoulos, S., Meyer, T. E., Conway, J. and Sleight, P. (1990) Effects of physical training on chronic heart failure. Lancet, 1, 63–66

Cohen, M. M. and Cameron, C. B. (1991) Should you cancel the operation when a child has an upper respiratory tract infection? Anesthesia and Analgesia, 72, 282–288

Coombs, D. W. (1983) Aspiration pneumonia prophylaxis. Anesthesia and Analgesia, 62, 1055–1058

Cote, C. J. (1990) NPO after midnight for children – a reappraisal. Anesthesiology, 72, 589–591

Dehring, D. J. and Arens, J. F. (1990) Pulmonary thromboembolism: disease recognition and patient management. Anesthesiology, 73, 146–164

Domar, A. D., Everett, L. L. and Keller, M. G. (1989) Preoperative anxiety: is it a predictable entity? Anesthesia and Analgesia, 69, 763–767

Dundee, J. W. and Fee, J. P. H. (1989) Nausea and vomiting after general anaesthesia. Lancet, 1, 1016

Editorial (1989a) Nausea and vomiting after general anaesthesia. Lancet, 1, 651–652

Editorial (1989b) Routine H2 receptor antagonists before elective surgery. Lancet, 1, 1363–1364

Edwards, R. (1985) Anaesthesia and alcohol. British Medical Journal, 2, 423–424

Egbert, L. D., Battit, G. E., Turndorf, H. and Beecher, H. K. (1963) The value of the preoperative visit by an anaesthetist. Journal of the American Medical Association, 185, 553–555

Egbert, L. D., Battit, G. E., Welch, C. E. and Bartlett, M. K. (1964) Reduction of postoperative pain by encouragement and instruction to the patient. New England Journal of Medicine, 270, 825–827

Endocarditis Working Party of the British Society for Antimicrobial Chemotherapy (1990) Antibiotic prophylaxis of infective endocarditis. Lancet, 1, 88–89

Evans, C. and Richardson, P. H. (1988) Improved recovery and reduced postoperative stay after therapeutic suggestions during general anaesthesia. Lancet, 2, 491–493

Fennelly, M. E. and Hall, G. M. (1990) Anaesthesia and upper respiratory tract infections. A non-existent hazard? British Journal of Anaesthesia, 64, 535–536

Goucke, C. R. (1989) Prophylaxis against venous thromboembolism. Anaesthesia and Intensive Care, 4, 58–65

Guillebaud, J. (1985) Surgery and the pill. British Medical Journal, 1, 498–499

Jones, R. M., Rosen, M. and Seymour, L. (1987) Smoking and anaesthesia. Anaesthesia, 42, 1–2

Joyce, T. H. 3rd (1987) Prophylaxis for pulmonary acid aspiration. American Journal of Medicine, 83 (Suppl 6A), 46–52

Leigh, J. M., Walker, J. and Janaganathan, P. (1977) Effect of preoperative anaesthetic visit on anxiety. British Medical Journal, 2, 987–989

Malins, A. F. (1978) Do they do as they are instructed? A review of outpatient anaesthesia. Anaesthesia, 33, 832–835

Maltby, J. R., Sutherland, A. D., Sale, J. P. and Shaffer, E. A. (1986) Preoperative oral fluids: is a five hour fast justified prior to elective surgery? Anesthesia and Analgesia, 65, 112–116

McCleane, G. J. and Cooper, R. (1990) The nature of pre-operative anxiety. *Anaesthesia*, **45**, 153–155

McLintock, T. T. C., Aitken, H., Downie, C. F. A. and Kenny, G. N. C. (1990) Postoperative analgesic requirements in patients exposed to positive intraoperative suggestions. *British Medical Journal*, **301**, 788–790

Miller, C. D. and Anderson, W. G. (1988) Silent regurgitation in day case gynaecological patients. *Anaesthesia*, **43**, 321–323

Miller, D. C. (1990) Why are children starved? *British Journal of Anaesthesia*, **64**, 409–410

Monroe, M. C., Gravenstein, N. and Saga-Rumley, S. (1990) Postoperative sore throat: effect of oropharyngeal airway in orotracheally intubated patients. *Anaesthesia and Analgesia*, **70**, 512–516

NHS Management Executive (1990) *A Guide to Consent for Examination or Treatment* (discussion paper)

Noone, P. (1988) Prophylactic use of antibiotics in surgery. *Hospital Update*, **14**, 1889–1896

Ong, B. Y., Palhniuk, R. J. and Cumming, M. (1978) Gastric volume and pH in out-patients. *Canadian Anaesthetists Society Journal*, **25**, 36–39

Pace, N. L. (1990) Prevention of succinylcholine myalgias: a meta-analysis. *Anesthesia and Analgesia*, **70**, 477–483

Palazzo, M. G. A. and Strunin, L. (1984a) Anaesthesia and emesis I: aetiology. *Canadian Anaesthetists Society Journal*, **31**, 178–187

Palazzo, M. G. A. and Strunin, L. (1984b) Anaesthesia and emesis II: prevention and management. *Canadian Anaesthetists Society Journal*, **31**, 407–415

Palmer, R. N. (1988) Consent and the anaesthetist. *Anaesthesia*, **43**, 265–266

Sandler, D. A. and Martin, J. F. (1989) Autopsy proven pulmonary embolism in hospital patients: are we detecting enough deep vein thrombosis? *Journal of the Royal Society of Medicine*, **82**, 203–205

Scarman, L. (1986) Consent, communication and responsibility. *Journal of the Royal Society of Medicine*, **79**, 697–700

Selsby, D. S. (1990) Chest physiotherapy; may be harmful in some patients. *British Medical Journal*, **1**, 541–542

Selsby, D. and Jones, J. G. (1990) Some physiological and clinical aspects of chest physiotherapy. *British Journal of Anaesthesia*, **64**, 621–633

Splinter, W. M., Stewart, J. A. and Muir, J. G. (1990) Large volumes of apple juice preoperatively do not affect gastric pH and volume in children. *Canadian Journal of Anaesthesia*, **37**, 36–39

Sprague, N. B. and Archer, P. L. (1987) Magill versus Mallinckrodt tracheal tubes. A comparative study of postoperative sore throat. *Anaesthesia*, **42**, 306–311

Stein, M. and Cassara, E. L. (1970) Preoperative pulmonary evaluation and therapy for surgery patients. *Journal of the American Medical Association*, **211**, 787–790

Sue-Ling, H. and Hughes, L. E. (1988) Should the pill be stopped pre-operatively? *British Medical Journal*, **1**, 447–448

Sutherland, A. D., Maltby, J. R., Sale, J. P. and Reid, C. R. G. (1987) The effect of preoperative oral fluid and ranitidine on gastric fluid volume and pH. *Canadian Journal of Anaesthesia*, **34**, 117–121

Tremper, K. K. and Barker, S. J. (1989) Pulse oximetry. *Anesthesiology*, **70**, 98–108

Whitehead, E. M. and Whitehead, M. I. (1991) The pill, HRT and post-operative thromboembolism: cause for concern? *Anaesthesia*, **46**, 521–522

# 4

# Care in the operating theatre

## Reception in theatre

It is customary for a member of the ward staff to bring patients to the operating theatre, so that they are accompanied by someone who is familiar to them. This nurse should be responsible for presenting the patient to the theatre nurse or anaesthetist who receives them. At this stage both the ward nurse and the theatre staff should satisfy themselves of the identity of the patient, and this may be done by checking the name and the hospital number of the patient from the operating list to the wrist band, and comparing them with the name and number on the notes and X-rays. A correctly signed consent form, with the operation to be performed clearly indicated, must be present, and again must agree with the published operating list. If the procedure is unilateral this should be stated on the form and be the same as that on the operating list. Ideally the side and site of the operation should also be marked on the patient.

It is vital that a designated person carries out this check and this is usually delegated to a member of the theatre nursing staff. The anaesthetist however must be sure that this has been done, either by observing the check, or by repeating it in person. If the anaesthetist already knows the patient because of a previous visit to the ward, then it is less likely that mistakes will happen. It is common practice in some hospitals to repeat the full preoperative ward check when the patient arrives in the operating theatre. At this time the patient will probably have received premedication, may not be fully alert and is often anxious. Further questioning will not provide theatre staff with satisfactory answers and it could be confusing or distressing to the patient. By the time the patient arrives in the anaesthetic room the anaesthetist should be familiar with the information needed before inducing anaesthesia. It is reasonable none the less to consult the notes to revise the patient's history and clinical examination, and to confirm the results of investigations ordered.

# Preparation in the operating theatre

Critical incidents are events that either lead to adverse outcome or would have led to such outcome if not detected. In anaesthetic practice about 50% of such incidents occur in the period from the time the patient enters the anaesthetic room until the induction of anaesthesia. Most incidents are due to human error and many are related to the equipment used. The most common equipment problems are breathing circuit disconnections, errors in gas flow and supply, and nonfunctioning laryngoscopes. Errors also occur in drug administration or labelling, and with disconnection or misplacement of intravenous infusions. The factors that contribute to these errors are inexperience, lack of familiarity with apparatus, poor communication and supervision, haste, carelessness, fatigue and inattention, and failure to perform adequate preoperative checks (Cooper, Newbower and Kitz, 1984).

## *Equipment*

All necessary equipment must be available and working correctly before anaesthesia is induced. There is no justification for an adverse patient outcome that is secondary to failure to perform a proper equipment check. Until recently it has not been customary for anaesthetists to observe a preset routine of apparatus checks before starting an anaesthetic. In the past few years a comparison has been made between this simplistic approach and the sophisticated preflight checks that are compulsory for airline pilots before take-off (Crosby, 1988), and some departments now require completion of a checklist before an operating room session starts. Introduction of such a checklist may contribute to a decrease in potential risk to patients (Kumar *et al.*, 1988), and the list can also be used as an *aide-mémoire* throughout the anaesthetic and recovery. Table 4.1 shows a suggested anaesthetic checklist. In its most structured form this involves the anaesthetist and an assistant reading through a list of items, confirming verbally and in writing for each item that the relevant procedure has been performed or control correctly set. Such formal compliance with preoperative checks ensures completeness in the process of preoperative preparation but is more rigorous than the checks that are generally applied at present. The value of a formal checklist has still to be proved. Compliance will be poor with one that is unreasonably detailed and it is necessary to define a simple, relevant procedure to be followed before an operating list, and before and during each individual anaesthetic.

**Table 4.1    An anaesthetic checklist**

PREOPERATIVE CHECK
*1.   Apparatus*
ventilator ...    vapour? filled? ...   line pressure ...
venting ...       pressure alarm ...
suction ...       mask ...   airways ...   ET tube ...
connector ...     stylet ...   laryngoscope ...

*2.   Lines*
i.v.   number? size? location?
?arterial

*3.   Monitors*
ECG, twitch, $CO_2$, $SpO_2$, N-G tube,
temp., urine

*4.   Drugs*
atropine ..., suxamethonium ...
antibiotics? DVT prophylaxis? resus.?
induction
relaxation
analgesia
volatiles, $N_2O$
Fluids: crystalloid, colloid, blood
**Patient allergy? ...**

*5.   Patient*
ID, consent,
Operation; side, position, warming blkt?
Postop; recovery, ICU
Airway; NPO, mouth opening, teeth (caps etc.)
Results;
Rapid sequence? Pre-oxygenation?
Protection: $H_2$-blocker, antacid, metoclopramide?

*6.   Ready to start?*
assistance


ANAESTHETIC ROOM
*1.   Before leaving*
pre-oxygenate, turn off gases, monitor


THEATRE
*1.   Connect patient*
gas and machine,
ventilator?

*2.   Check patient*
warm, pink, capillary refill, breathing

*3.   Check monitors and alarms*
attached, working, alarms

*4.   OK for surgery?*
ETT position, connection, fixation
eyes closed, protected
thorax and abdomen free
joints, pressure points, nerves
access to lines + tubing

RELIEF CHECK
1.  *Patient*
ID, operation, relevant problems

2.  *Anaesthesia*
induction, maintenance, relaxants due?
analgesia due?
fluids
surgical course
anaesthetic course
problems intraop?
where to contact

PROGNOSIS
expected problems
expected info (investigations etc.)

**Completed by:**

NAME . . . . . . . . . . . . . . . . .   DATE . . . . . . . . .   TIME . . . . . . . . .

---

*Anaesthetic machine*

The anaesthetic machine should be completely checked before the beginning of each list. The Association of Anaesthetists of Great Britain and Ireland has published its recommendations for an anaesthetic machine checklist (Association of Anaesthetists ..., 1990) and a summary is given in Table 4.2. In the United Kingdom the anaesthetic machine is usually connected and tested by an anaesthetic technician before an operating session. This does not relieve the anaesthetist of the responsibility for checking the machine, and this should be performed by the anaesthetist, either alone or working with an assistant, at the beginning of each operating session. The checklist given in Table 4.2 may not fully apply to all anaesthetic machines, and changes in design and technology will undoubtedly mean that revisions will be necessary at a later date. The recommendations state that a record should be kept of the checks performed, either in a specific logbook for each anaesthetic machine, or by an entry in the patient's anaesthetic chart.

The first part of the check is to inspect the machine for obvious damage or faults and to check and connect the antipollution system. The oxygen analyser is then fitted and calibrated and the medical gas supply and vaporizers are checked. A suitable breathing system must be connected to the machine and confirmation made that it functions properly, and where a ventilator is to be used this must also be checked and shown to be working correctly. Suction is necessary whenever and wherever any anaesthetic is administered, and the system must be checked to see whether adequate negative pressure is generated, and to confirm that a selection of rigid and flexible suction catheters to connect to the system are available. Much equipment requires an electrical power source and it is important that all such monitors and alarms are turned on before the start of the anaesthetic, warmed up where necessary, and properly calibrated. Appropriate levels will need to be set on the alarms.

**Table 4.2** **Suggested machine check based on Association of Anaesthetists recommendations (1990)**

**1. Inspection**

(a) Inspect machine for damage to flowmeters, vaporizers, gauges and hoses. Check all flowmeters off, cylinders off, vaporizers off. Cylinder key available. Note date of last service. If unfamiliar machine, check which safety devices and alarms are installed. If breathing system or ventilator unfamiliar seek instruction or change it.
(b) Check antipollution system. Connect to machine

**2. Oxygen analyser**

(a) Check and calibrate to monitor gases leaving common gas outlet

**3. Medical gas supplies**

(a) Disconnect all pipelines. Electrical supply on
(b) Check cylinders present, securely seated and off. Carbon dioxide cylinder should not normally be left on the machine
(c) Open flowmeter control valves
(d) Turn on reserve oxygen cylinder and check contents and oxygen flow through flowmeter. Repeat test if there is a second oxygen cylinder
Check oxygen flow control valve can adjust flow over full range of flowmeter and set flow for approximately 5 l/min
Oxygen analyser display should not vary significantly from 100%
(e) Turn on reserve nitrous oxide cylinder and check contents and nitrous oxide flow through flowmeter. Repeat test if there is a second nitrous oxide cylinder
Check nitrous oxide flow control valve can adjust flow over full range of flowmeter and set flow for approximately 5 l/min
(f) Turn off oxygen cylinder(s) and empty oxygen from the system with the oxygen flush valve. Cylinder gauge should return to zero. Audible oxygen alarm should sound while oxygen pressure is decreasing. When oxygen supply fails confirm appropriate oxygen failure protection device functions to prevent delivery of hypoxic gas mixture
(g) Connect oxygen pipeline. This should restore flow of oxygen and cancel the oxygen failure protection device. Perform 'tug' test and check oxygen pipeline pressure reads 400 kPa
(h) Turn off nitrous oxide cylinder(s). Connect nitrous oxide pipeline. This should restore flow of nitrous oxide through nitrous oxide flowmeter. Perform 'tug' test and check nitrous oxide pipeline pressure reads 400 kPa. Turn off nitrous oxide flowmeter control valve
(i) If other cylinders are required these should also be checked in a similar way
(j) Turn off all flowmeter control valves
(k) Operate energency oxygen flush valve and ensure that there is no significant decrease in pipline pressure. Confirm that oxygen analyser reads close to 100%

### 4. Vaporizers

(a) Check that vaporizer(s) for required agent(s) are fitted correctly, that any backbar locking mechanism is fully engaged, and that control knob(s) rotate through their full range(s). Turn off vaporizer(s)
(b) Check that flow through any vaporizer is in the correct direction
(c) When filling vaporizer ensure correct anaesthetic agent is used, and that filling port is left tightly closed
(d) Where an anaesthetic machine is fitted with a pressure relief valve the following test should be performed:
  (i) Set test flow (6–8 l/min) and with the vaporizer off temporarily occlude common gas outlet. There should be no leak from any vaporizer fitments and the flowmeter bobbin will dip
  (ii) Repeat the test with the vaporizer in the on position. There should be no leak from the filling port. Turn off the vaporizer(s) and the oxygen flowmeter control valve

### 5. Breathing systems

(a) Inspect the configuration of the breathing and scavenging systems and check they function correctly. Ensure there are no leaks or obstructions
(b) The 'push and twist' technique should be employed for connecting conical fittings.
(c) Check the adjustable pressure limiting 'expiratory' valve can be fully opened and closed. Leave in an open position
(d) With Bain circuits perform a visual check and an occlusion test on the inner tube. With circle systems check the function of unidirectional valves, freshness of soda lime, leave expiratory valve open and soda lime in circuit

### 6. Ventilator

(a) Check normal operation of the ventilator and its controls
(b) Occlude the patient port and check the pressure relief valve functions correctly
(c) Check the disconnect alarm is present and operational
(d) Ensure there is an alternative means to ventilate the patient's lungs in the event of ventilator malfunction

### 7. Suction equipment

(a) Check all components and test that an adequate negative pressure is generated

### 8. Electrical equipment

(a) Turned on, warmed up, calibrated

### 9. Alarms

(a) Turn on and set appropriate alarms

### Rapid check

This may be used before each case and in emergency situations

1. Check that the flowmeters are off
2. Check that the vaporizers are sufficiently full and turned off
3. Check that the cylinder contents are sufficient and pipeline pressures normal
4. Check that the breathing system is complete and correctly assembled, that the connections are tight and leak-free, and that the soda lime is not exhausted
5. Check that suction is available, working to normal vacuum and within reach

## Other equipment

*Anaesthetic equipment*   The equipment needed for performing mask anaesthesia and endotracheal intubation in adults is listed in Table 4.3, but additional equipment, tube sizes etc. will sometimes be required. Some of the equipment required for paediatric anaesthesia is specialized and should be readily available from a separate dedicated paediatric box or trolley. Masks, airways and tubes should be checked for patency and it should be ensured that all connectors are compatible. The commonest endotracheal tube size for an adult male is 9 mm internal diameter and 8 mm for an adult female. It is normal British practice to precut the tubes, in which case for an oral tube a length of 23 cm is appropriate for a male and 21 cm for a female. The cuff on the tube should be inflated to test for leaks. At least two laryngoscopes with appropriate blades giving adequate illumination should be present.

**Table 4.3   Essential anaesthetic equipment for adults**

*Airway and intubation*
1. Masks – sizes 3–5
2. Airways – oral sizes 2–4. Nasopharyngeal sizes 6.0–8.0
3. Laryngoscopes (2) with a selection of blades
4. Endotracheal tubes 6.0–9.0, laryngeal mask airways
5. Syringe for cuff inflation
6. Clamp to seal cuff tubing if valve not included
7. Suction – with rigid and flexible suction catheters

*Aids to intubation*
8. Introducers and bougies
9. Magill's forceps

*I.V. therapy*
10. Intravenous cannulae, administration sets, fluid

*Emergency drugs and equipment*
11. Failed intubation apparatus; emergency cricothyrotomy set, emergency tracheostomy set, fibreoptic intubating bronchoscope
12. Resuscitation drugs
13. Defibrillator

The possibility of a difficult intubation must always be anticipated and at each anaesthetic location there should be a selection of laryngoscope blades, bougies and introducers to aid with intubation and, as a last resort, an emergency cricothyroidotomy set. Additional equipment is usefully assembled on a 'difficult intubation trolley', which will carry an emergency tracheostomy set and a wider range of tubes, airways, introducers, masks, laryngeal masks and, where the trained staff are available, a fibreoptic intubating bronchoscope and a rigid bronchoscope. A resuscitation trolley must be sited near every anaesthetic location. This should carry a defibrillator and resuscitation drugs. This trolley must be regularly checked, and be easy to access in a known and open location.

*Additional equipment*    The anaesthetist may also require other pieces of equipment which are for the benefit of the patient but whose use reflects the duration, nature and extent of the procedure rather than direct anaesthetic requirements. Such equipment includes nasogastric tubes, heat and moisture exchangers, blood warmers and warming coils, warming blankets and pressure infusers.

## Monitors

Monitors should be available in the anaesthetic room and the operating theatres, connected to the correct power supply, calibrated and warmed up if necessary. See Chapter 5 for a full discussion and details of minimum monitoring.

## Intravascular cannulae

A range of intravenous cannulae must be available. The flow of fluid through a cannula is related to the fourth power of the radius and a cannula of 16 gauge or greater should therefore be inserted if fluid resuscitation or blood administration is necessary. To prevent disconnection all cannulae should be attached via a Luer–Lok type of connector to a cap, fluid administration set or manometer line. At present there is no standard colour coding for intravenous cannulae in the United Kingdom, although moves to establish one are under way (Tordoff and Sweeney, 1990).

Central venous placement of lines calls for an additional range of cannulae. In the United Kingdom it is still common to use long over-needle cannulae for this purpose, although the use of catheter over guide wire (Seldinger technique) cannulae is increasing, especially when more than one central line is required.

## Drugs

A full range of anaesthetic and resuscitation drugs should be kept in the operating theatre and be available when required. A more limited stock should be closer to hand in the anaesthetic room. It is the responsibility of the anaesthetist to ensure that the patient receives the correct drug in the right dosage. In most hospitals the nursing practice is for two nurses to check a drug and dosage before administration, but this is not the routine in anaesthetic practice, the doctor taking sole responsibility. Thus when drawing up a drug great care must be taken to ensure the correct dosage, and that the syringe into which the drug has been withdrawn is clearly labelled. The responsibility for this can be delegated to a colleague or a qualified assistant. In these circumstances it is necessary to be certain that no confusion arises over the drug or dosage contained in the syringe. The anaesthetist remains responsible for all drugs given while he or she is in control of the patient and must therefore be confident of the contents of syringes. Errors, sometimes resulting in serious injury or death, have occurred when incorrect drugs or dosage have been administered. In some hospitals a supply of anaesthetic drugs, especially those used for emergency obstetric anaesthesia, are drawn up, labelled and left in a safe place. This practice cannot be condoned as it is unusual not to have time to draw up fresh anaesthetic agents, and it is obviously a system that can easily lead to errors. If this practice is allowed, the drugs drawn up should be clearly marked with the name of the person who drew them up, and the time and date at which this was done. It should be remembered that there is always the possibility that unattended drugs may be stolen or tampered with. If the contents of a syringe cannot be ascertained with confidence the only safe rule is to discard the drug to ensure that a patient does not receive it. Any drugs unused at the end of a procedure should be destroyed, and the syringe and needle disposed of in a suitable container.

Ampoules of drugs are supplied in packets which usually include a leaflet containing valuable information describing the agent and the dosage. The labelling of the actual ampoules is nonstandard, often difficult to read, confusing and potentially dangerous. Widely different products are sometimes labelled in a similar way, and it is therefore easy to draw up the wrong drug or concentration unless care is exercised at all times. Several cases with fatal outcome to patients have been reported where potassium chloride solution was used to dissolve drugs instead of saline. Pharmacies may change drug suppliers and, as there is no uniformity in labelling of drugs by the manufacturers, confusing changes in packaging and presentation are common.

Size, colouring and lettering of drug labels provided for syringes may differ between hospitals or even within the same hospital. Standards for labelling have been formulated for the United States and mistakes might be avoided if similar measures were adopted in the United Kingdom. The United States specification proposed by the American Society for Testing and Materials (ASTM) is outlined in Table 4.4. The proposals lay down standards for what the label should say, and for the size, legibility and orientation of the lettering on the label.

There must be few anaesthetists who have not, at some time, administered the wrong drug, or wrong dose of a drug, to a patient. In order to minimize this possibility it is advisable to limit the number of drugs that are drawn up, to routinely use a certain size of syringe

Table 4.4    ASTM label recommendations

1. Contents
   Generic name of drug
   Amount of drug per unit
   Acceptable abbreviations

2. Size
   As large as possible (10 point or larger preferred)

3. Orientation
   Print parallel to long axis of container unless the name and amount of drug can
   be printed within 180° around the circumference of the container, in which case
   the copy may be perpendicular to the long axis of the container

4. Legibility
   Provide contrast between the type used for information and the drug container
   or background of the label. The name and amount of drug per unit should be
   legible in a light of 215 lux at a distance of 500 mm by a person with 20 : 20 vision

In addition each group of drugs is identified by a distinct colour, e.g. yellow for
induction agents, red for muscle relaxants, blue for narcotics, green for parasym-
pathetics

---

for a selected drug, and where possible to have a set routine for the
placement and storage of drugs in the operating theatre. As an example,
thiopentone can always be drawn up into a 20 ml syringe and the
nondepolarizing muscle relaxant into a 5 ml syringe. At the end of a
procedure avoid the risk of inadvertently giving a muscle relaxant
instead of the neuromuscular antagonist by discarding the relaxant
before drawing up the antagonist.

*Emergency drugs*

It is common practice in some hospitals to have an ampoule of
suxamethonium and atropine drawn up and available for every case.
Although there are undoubtedly times when these drugs are urgently
needed this practice is expensive and wasteful, and might lead to the
wrong drug being given. It is, however, essential that resuscitation
drugs are immediately available, and the supply of some drugs in a
prepacked syringe form is one method of achieving this without the
need to open unwanted ampoules.

The anaesthetic area must contain drugs that may be required to
manage respiratory and cardiovascular problems occurring in anaesthetized patients. For airway and respiratory problems these drugs
include suxamethonium to provide neuromuscular blockade of rapid
onset, and adrenaline, hydrocortisone and nebulized and intravenous
salbutamol to treat bronchospasm. Vasoconstrictors such as ephedrine
or phenylephrine, and vasodilators such as labetalol are used regularly
during routine anaesthesia, while other inotropes, vasopressors and

vasodilators are given, usually by infusion, in more specialized circumstances. An anticholinergic, such as atropine, is often required to prevent or treat a bradycardia, whereas a tachycardia under anaesthesia usually requires fluid resuscitation or an increase in depth of anaesthesia. If dysrhythmias occur, provocative factors such as hypoxia, hypercarbia, the use of halothane, light anaesthesia and intense surgical stimulation must first of all be excluded before resorting to the use of antidysrhythmics such as lignocaine. The first line treatment of severe anaphylactoid reactions is adrenaline, and this must always be available. For acute emergencies such as severe anaphylactoid reactions, cardiac arrest or collapse, it is important to have a resuscitation box containing all the immediately necessary drugs.

It is worth noting that when immediate intravenous access is not available, atropine, lignocaine, adrenaline and other drugs that do not cause tissue damage are effective when administered by the intratracheal route in a dose of 1–2 times the intravenous dose diluted in 10 ml of sterile water. Sodium bicarbonate and calcium for resuscitation must not be given intratracheally as they will damage the mucosa and alveoli.

## Opioids

Because of the potential for abuse it is particularly important to control the use of potent analgesic drugs. They should be allocated on a named patient basis, not left lying unattended in theatres or anaesthetic rooms, and any surplus must be destroyed or handed back at the end of the anaesthetic session.

In the United Kingdom the Misuse of Drugs Act 1971 empowers the Secretary of State to provide for the safe custody of controlled drugs and the keeping of records of their prescription. The Misuse of Drugs Regulations 1985 define who is authorized to supply and possess controlled drugs while acting in a professional capacity, and lay down the conditions under which these activities may be carried out. In these regulations the drugs are divided into five schedules each specifying the requirements governing activities such as production, supply, possession, prescribing and record keeping which apply to them. The administration of opioids such as pethidine, morphine and fentanyl is regulated by Schedule 2. The Duthie Report on 'the guidelines for the safe and secure handling of medicines' suggests rules to ensure the safety and security of medicines stored and used in the operating department. An appointed nurse is responsible for the secure storage and control of the controlled drug stock, including recording the amount issued to medical staff in a controlled drug record. The anaesthetist must sign for drugs received, record the amount administered on the anaesthetic chart, return unopened ampoules to the apointed nurse, and safely dispose of unused medicines.

## Assistance

An anaesthetic should not be administered unless trained and competent assistance is available to the anaesthetist. The assistant must be present at induction, and be available throughout the procedure. A skilled and attentive assistant undoutedly contributes to the safety and efficiency of anaesthesia. In the United Kingdom the anaesthetist is fortunate to be able to rely on excellent operating department assistants (ODA) or anaesthetic nurses for assistance. They prepare the anaesthetic induction room and operating theatre for the anaesthetic, and assist the anaesthetist with his work. They should be able to anticipate most of the requirements of the anaesthetist for a given procedure and procure and set up such equipment, monitors, lines etc. that will be needed. They also help with checking the anaesthetic machine and procuring drugs. During induction and other times of activity when the anaesthetist may not be able to observe the patient continuously as closely as is desirable, the assistant provides an extra pair of trained eyes and ears with which to monitor the patient. Because these assistants know the layout of the operating theatres, their help is invaluable in emergency situations when drugs and equipment are urgently required by an anaesthetist who is fully committed to caring directly for the patient.

# Induction

Induction can only begin after the checks and preparations detailed above have been carried out.

## Place of induction

### Induction in an anaesthetic room

It is common British practice to induce anaesthesia in a room adjoining the operating theatre, and several advantages are claimed for this practice. The room is an area which the anaesthetist can control, containing space to store drugs and equipment. To be taken from a ward bed and placed directly on an operating table is a frightening experience for patients, whereas the anaesthetic room should provide a quiet, calm haven away from the noise and bustle of the operating theatre and the comments of surgeons and theatre staff, where the anaesthetist is obviously in charge. There are particular advantages for children as it is reasonable for parents to remain in the anaesthetic room until anaesthesia is induced. If there is a delay before the induction starts, the anaesthetic room provides a suitable waiting area for the patient and escort nurse. Drugs and equipment can be made ready for the patient and the anaesthetic assistant can make preliminary preparations by carrying out some checks and attaching monitors. If two anaesthetists are engaged on the list, then anaesthesia can be induced in the anaesthetic room while the previous operation is completed. More complex anaesthetics often require considerable preparation, for example the insertion of an epidural catheter or the placement of central venous lines or a pulmonary artery flotation catheter. In these cases valuable time can be saved between operations by utilizing the anaesthetic room while the operating theatre is still occupied.

## Induction in the operating theatre

Although in the United Kingdom induction usually takes place in a separate anaesthetic room, there is a considerable body of opinion that believes that, at least in some cases, this should be performed in the operating theatres with the patient already positioned on the operating table. In many countries it is the routine practice to induce anaesthesia in this way. If anaesthesia is regularly started in the operating theatres then arrangements can be made to store vital equipment close at hand or on trolleys that are wheeled in when needed. Good practice, reinforced by the published minimum monitoring standards of the professional anaesthetic organizations, dictates that vital signs should be continuously monitored in all patients from the induction of anaesthesia until recovery is assured, and this is especially important if patients are seriously ill or cardiovascularly unstable. It is expensive to provide two complete sets of adequate monitors both in the anaesthetic room and the operating theatre, and the process of disconnection and reconnection of monitoring is time-consuming and dangerous, diverting attention from the patient at the very time when full monitoring is needed. If anaesthesia is induced in the operating theatres then monitoring can be attached before induction and observed continuously thereafter. The same consideration applies when using two anaesthetic machines and circuits where disconnection and reconnection of the patient's airway must complicate the procedure and increase risks.

There is no real evidence to suggest that patients suffer greatly increased anxiety when induced in the operating theatre rather than the anaesthetic room, and it is routine, even in the United Kingdom, for many seriously ill patients to be anaesthetized in this way. As one case cannot be started until the previous one has finished, this system gives greater opportunity for a senior anaesthetist to supervise the work of a trainee. It is also possible that wider use of this practice would enable surgeons to gain a better appreciation of the skills required and the time that is needed to anaesthetize a patient and prepare for surgery.

Many day care units do not have anaesthetic rooms, and thus patients anaesthetized there are induced in the operating theatres. Patients are often unpremedicated and are able to walk into the operating room and be assisted on to the operating table. Little preparation is necessary and the routine monitoring can be easily and swiftly attached prior to induction. This system speeds up turnover of cases and ensures that the patients are adequately monitored even though the procedures may be brief.

## Non-medical staff at induction

### Parents accompanying children

Many parents express the wish to bring their child to theatre and be present at the start of the anaesthetic (Hannallah and Rosales, 1983; Schofield and White, 1989). The most important consideration must be whether there is any benefit to the child. The parent, a sure reference point for the child, may be able to calm fears, provide assurance and aid compliance during the rather frightening procedures accompanying anaesthesia. If the child remains asleep during induction of anaesthesia the presence of the parent is less useful. Heavy premedication should not be a substitute for proper preoperative explanation to, and preparation of, the parent and child. Watching a child being anaesthetized is a distressing experience for any parent and sometimes this generates anxieties which can be transmitted to the child. In these circumstances the presence of the parent is detrimental. The overriding consideration is that the parent should not interfere with the safe conduct of the anaesthetic, and it should therefore be made clear to parents that they must leave immediately if asked to do so. Some anaesthetists, especially if they are inexperienced, or if the child is unwell or the operation a major procedure, may find that the parent is a distracting influence and in these cases it will be better for the patient if the parent is not present at induction. Although some pressure groups, often with medical support, strongly advocate that a parent should always be present at induction of anaesthesia, the final decision must rest with the anaesthetist in the best interests of the patient. There can be no departure from this rule and it should be made clear to all concerned from the outset.

In summary, the influence of the parents is usually beneficial, while the administration of a well-conducted anaesthetic should be open to scrutiny and is unlikely to cause undue alarm in most adults. Parents, if they so request, should therefore generally be allowed to accompany their children up to the time of induction.

*Anaesthesia in the presence of the spouse*

It is now acceptable common practice for husbands to be present during delivery by caesarean section performed under a regional block, and many will stay for the duration of labour and thus see the placement of the epidural catheter and the commencement of regional anaesthesia. The husband can provide support to his wife and shares the experience of being present at the birth of the child. There is now increasing pressure for husbands to be present during caesarean sections performed under a general anaesthetic (Bogod, 1990), partly out of concern over reports of mothers being given the wrong baby. This is generally less acceptable and must be at the discretion of the anaesthetist.

## Pre-oxygenation

Pre-oxygenating patients before induction of anaesthesia increases arterial oxygenation ($PaO_2$) and delays the fall in oxygen saturation that will result if there is any difficulty with ventilation immediately after induction (Gould, 1989). Pre-oxygenation should be performed in any patient with potential airway or ventilation problems, before a rapid sequence induction of anaesthesia, or in old, sick or obese patients. It is especially important in operative obstetrics. The traditional technique has been to ask the patient to breathe 100% oxygen for 3 minutes or longer at normal tidal volumes. However, four vital capacity breaths over 30 seconds will probably be as effective. With a rapid induction technique pre-oxygenation is preferable to ventilation with oxygen after paralysis is achieved as this prevents inflation of the stomach which increases the risk of regurgitation. It is important to realize that adequate pre-oxygenation is so effective that a patient who receives no further oxygen may not be noticeably hypoxic for perhaps as long as 10 minutes. Thus the danger is that an oesophageal intubation or other cause of failure to oxygenate may remain undiscovered until cyanosis is seen or the oxygen saturation falls, and this may be after surgery has begun. The placement of the endotracheal tube must be suspect in these circumstances.

# The difficult airway

## The obstructed airway

The major cause of mortality and severe morbidity attributable to anaesthesia is the result of inability to secure the airway in order to allow unobstructed respiration. Great care must be used when inducing general anaesthesia unless the anaesthetist is confident that the patient's airway can be maintained. Anatomical and pathological factors determine whether it will be possible to maintain a patent airway in the anaesthetized patient and difficulties can be expected in patients with tumours or trauma in and around the head and neck. If the patient breathes normally when awake it is rare, but by no means unknown, for it to be very difficult or impossible to maintain the airway under general anaesthesia. In order to maintain a patent airway it is often necessary to pull the mandible forward and to use aids such as oral or nasal airways. Mechanical ventilation with a bag and mask is often more difficult than maintaining an airway with the patient breathing spontaneously. Where difficulties are anticipated paralysing agents should, in general, not be used until the ability to ventilate the patient's lungs has been confirmed. If an endotracheal tube can be placed successfully the airway will be secured, but this is often more difficult than using a mask and airway to ensure unobstructed respiration.

## The difficult intubation

Successful endotracheal intubation results in a clear airway which is isolated from gastric contents. It is not always easy to be certain that the tube is correctly placed, and unrecognized oesophageal intubation is an important cause of mortality and major morbidity. It is necessary to understand that auscultatory confirmation of proper endotracheal tube placement is often misleading (Caplan et al., 1990). A difficult and prolonged intubation is also associated with the risk of hypoxia. If a difficult intubation is anticipated as a result of a preoperative visit, a decision can be taken, after discussion with the patient, either to use an anaesthetic technique that does not require intubation, or to use one of the methods designed to overcome the difficulty. Intubating an awake patient preserves protective airway reflexes, is not difficult to learn and is well tolerated. A skilled operator can usually intubate with the aid of a fibreoptic bronchoscope, either with the patient awake or asleep. Because of the preparation time required, and the difficulties in visualization after trauma has caused bleeding in the pharynx, where the necessary expertise and equipment are available, this technique should probably be considered the method of choice. It should not be reserved for use when other methods have failed. Many other techniques have been described, including blind nasal intubation, passing a tube over a guide inserted retrogradely through the cricothyroid membrane, and the use of a light wand to identify the larynx.

Although several methods have been devised in an attempt to predict which patients will be difficult to intubate (Mallampati et al., 1985; Samsoon and Young, 1987), the apparently normal subject can unexpectedly prove to be a problem. Thus all anaesthetists must be prepared to deal with a difficult or failed intubation (Vaughan, 1989) by employing a 'failed intubation drill', such as that suggested by Tunstall (1976). The various techniques mentioned above can be used to achieve intubation in these circumstances, but none of them is totally reliable and all require considerable skill. The cardinal lesson to note is that patients die from a failure of oxygenation, not from a failure to intubate. Oxygenation must be maintained during attempts at intubation and if this cannot be achieved with a face mask then an emergency cricothyroidotomy provides a quick method of providing temporary ventilation, although it provides no protection against soiling of the airway (Safar and Pennickx, 1967; Boyce and Peters, 1989). The laryngeal mask airway (LMA, Brain airway) may be used to maintain an airway and allow the operation to proceed when intubation proves impossible (Calder et al., 1990). The LMA provides inadequate protection against gastric aspiration and it is not a substitute for intubation with a cuffed endotracheal tube in patients likely to regurgitate.

The LMA can also be an aid to intubation in cases of difficulty. It may be possible to pass a 6.0 mm tube through the LMA directly into the trachea (Heath and Allagain, 1990), or the LMA may aid placement of a gum elastic bougie over which the endotracheal tube can be passed (Allison and McCrory, 1990). The LMA also makes fibreoptic intubation very easy, although this is a complicated method for placing an endotracheal tube.

## Intravascular access

In most patients there is no difficulty in gaining venous access. Intravenous access not only provides the usual route for induction of anaesthesia, but is the best route by which emergency drugs can be given for resuscitation if they become necessary. If induction of anaesthesia by the intravenous route is to be employed then a safe, secure and reliable access should be obtained prior to induction. In some patients this may be technically very difficult whereas, under the influence of a general anaesthetic, vasodilatation occurs so that it then becomes possible to insert a large cannula easily into a vein. In these circumstances a small cannula can usually be placed to gain adequate venous access for safe induction and it can then be replaced if necessary with a larger cannula once the patient is asleep. Only rarely is it impossible to find a vein in an awake patient and the patient then has to have an inhalational induction with insertion of the venous cannula once anaesthetized. If placing a peripheral line is not possible but venous access is considered essential to the safety of the patient, then a central venous line should be inserted before induction of anaesthesia, or a surgical cut-down employed.

## Problems from intravascular access

### Intravenous access

There are many complications of peripheral intravenous injections and from the fluids given in this way, some resulting in considerable discomfort for the patient, although permanent sequelae are rare. Thrombophlebitis is the commonest result and it can be minimized by avoiding small veins whenever possible and by flushing through the cannula with physiological saline after the administration of each dose of drug. The reported incidence of thrombophlebitis from a continuous infusion varies widely but is commonly greater than 50% (Lewis and Hecker, 1985; Hecker, 1989). Many factors are involved, of which the most important are the duration of infusion, the drugs used, and the nature of the solutions infused. There is some evidence that the type and size of the cannulae contribute, and the use of certain materials is more likely to cause damage to the intima of the vessel. Anaesthetic induction agents are generally irritant and may cause phlebitis; of the intravenous agents, diazepam is particularly prone to do this. The incidence of thrombophlebitis may be reduced by adding heparin or hydrocortisone to the infusion, by changing infusion sites regularly, and by avoiding solutions with a low pH. Nitroglycerine patches placed near the insertion site have been shown to prolong the life of a drip, presumably by causing local vasodilatation.

Serious damage can occur if certain drugs are allowed to extravasate into tissue instead of being injected into a vein. The solutions especially likely to cause problems from extravascular injection are calcium, potassium and sodium bicarbonate, and any that are hypertonic such as strong dextrose solution, mannitol and urea. Metal needles are particularly likely to cut out of the vein, and the injection site should be closely watched as the injection is given; great care must be exercised when repeated injections are to be given. Cytotoxic drugs should never be given in this way.

The doctor initiating an intravenous infusion should specify to the nurse in charge a regime for its care, including regular inspection of all cannulation sites. If there is a suspicion that the cannula has tissued it should be flushed carefully with saline to check the placement, and if there is any doubt it must be removed and resited.

### Inadvertent arterial injection

The arteries are extremely susceptible to damage from solutions that are not isotonic or of the correct pH. Great care must be exercised to avoid accidental injection into an artery, by palpation for pulsation when inserting a line or making an injection, and by observation of the colour and flow of blood withdrawn at initial cannulation. An isolated injection of a drug into the brachial artery can occur when needles or cannulae are placed in the cubital fossa, although care must also be taken to avoid the radial and ulnar arteries when injections are made in the wrist area. Most drugs cause pain when injected into an artery and result in intense spasm of the vessel followed by thrombosis and loss of the distal blood supply. Immediate treatment when this is suspected consists of injection of procaine and papaverine into the artery to relieve pain and promote vasodilatation. Later treatment includes anticoagulation to prevent thrombosis, and a local sympathetic block, to maintain the vasodilatation.

## Insertion of lines

In addition to a peripheral venous line, it may be necessary to insert arterial, central venous or pulmonary arterial lines for patient monitoring and intravascular access. As with all invasive procedures, there are risks to the patient from these lines and these should be considered when a decision is made to place them. It is possible to insert all these lines under local anaesthesia prior to the induction of anaesthesia and this has the advantage that monitoring can be started before induction, an important consideration in seriously ill patients with cardiovascular instability. It may be that placing lines in the awake patient reduces the overall anaesthetic time, although few patients will benefit markedly from this. In some centres it is routine to insert lines in this way and it does not seem to increase patient anxiety unduly or have an affect on the complication rate. Many anaesthetists, however, prefer to place invasive monitoring lines after induction because this is quicker and less traumatic, for both patient and anaesthetist. While the anaesthetist is concentrating on inserting lines it is important that the patient's condition is monitored by an assistant.

All cannulations must be performed in a clean manner but it is essential that central venous cannulation is performed using an aseptic technique. This means that the anaesthetist should wash his or her hands, put on sterile gloves, clean the insertion site with an appropriate solution, and use sterile towels to protect the operative area from contamination. Long cannulae inserted over the needle are still commonly used in the United Kingdom to achieve central venous access. They are cheap and, in skilled hands, easy and quick to insert with a no-touch technique. The alternative is to use a catheter over a guide wire (Seldinger) technique, and this is probably safer as the narrower, shorter needle used for primary puncture is less likely to damage major vessels or cause a pneumothorax. With this technique multi-lumen catheters can be inserted with one puncture which must also minimize the risk of insertion when several central lines are needed. Several routes can be used to insert the central line and the techniques, indications and complications are well described elsewhere (Kaplan,

1979). Cannulations of the cubital fossa veins (basilic or cephalic) with a long cannula, and the external jugular vein with the aid of 'J-wire', carry a lower success for successful central placement than other routes but are associated with few major complications. When learning a technique of central cannulation the internal jugular route is associated with a lower incidence of pneumothorax than the subclavian route but has the risk of carotid artery puncture. Where a difficult internal jugular cannulation is anticipated the vein can be identified with little risk using a small needle before a larger needle is inserted.

Arterial cannulation allows direct, continuous measurement of arterial blood pressure and wave form analysis, and also facilitates collection of blood samples for measurement of arterial blood gases and other investigations. Several arteries are suitable but the radial artery is probably the most frequently used for intraoperative purposes. The pros and cons of various cannulation sites are well documented and one often-stated contraindication to radial cannulation is the presence of inadequate collateral circulation to the hand. It is usually suggested that this is assessed with the Allen test (Allen, 1929), although there is little evidence to demonstrate that this test is useful in predicting when arterial cannulation is of harm (Slogoff, Keats and Arlund, 1983). It should be noted that the brachial artery has no collateral circulation and the axillary artery, although not a first choice, is a satisfactory site for placement of an arterial line (see Chapter 5).

### Intravenous access before regional anaesthesia

It is advisable that intravenous access is obtained before starting a regional local anaesthetic block. Access is necessary to combat hypotension that may result from the block and for resuscitation should an overdose be given inadvertently or an adverse reaction be caused by the local anaesthetic. A sympathetic nervous system blockade, most commonly from a spinal or epidural anaesthetic, will cause vasodilatation in the area affected. Not only may this result in a drop in blood pressure but the compensatory vasoconstriction in the unaffected upper limbs may make inserting a cannula more difficult. It is advisable in these circumstances to use a large bore cannula since it may be necessary to give an infusion at a fast rate.

## The anaesthetized patient

An anaesthetized patient is unable to do anything but remain in the position and on the support on which he or she is placed. Vital protective reflexes are abolished and the patient can not indicate discomfort or pain, or take preventative action if harm is threatened. The anaesthetist must therefore take responsibility for preventing physical damage and this requires an appreciation of the problems that can occur and an attention to detail in preparing, positioning and looking after the anaesthetized patient.

## Moving and positioning the patient

It is obviously important to take care when moving and positioning an anaesthetized patient. Under anaesthesia muscles relax, and it is possible to place the patient in a position that would not easily be assumed in the awake state, and which may result in damage to nerve, vessel or other tissue. Once the patient has been covered with sterile towels it is difficult to check proper positioning and often impossible to make alterations to it, and it is therefore vital for the anaesthetist to be satisfied with the placement of the patient on the operating table before surgery begins. If patients are placed on the operating table in a potentially unstable position, such as on their side, they must be carefully supervised until they are secured in that position. The same close supervision is necessary whenever there is a possibility that the patient may suddenly move and fall from the table or bed, for example when recovering from the anaesthetic at the end of surgery.

Relaxation of protective musculature combined with the supine position and a hard, flat operating table commonly result in backache. This may be exacerbated by the use of the lithotomy position which increases rotation of the pelvis. Both legs must be lifted together when this position is adopted to prevent undue strain on the pelvic ligaments. The head, trunk and limbs must always be supported in a comfortable position. It is especially important to avoid undue extension or flexion of the neck, and this can occur if the prone position is adopted. Direct pressure can cause damage to soft tissues, especially in areas overlying bony points or to vulnerable areas such as the eyes, nose and ears. Poor tissue perfusion from low cardiac output or hypothermia make damage more likely. Improper application of a face mask or catheter mount can cause facial nerve injury, damage to eyebrows, eyes and the bridge of the nose. Heels should be protected by supports placed under the ankles and other areas at risk padded with cotton wool or similar material. Care must be taken to ensure that the corneas do not become dry or injured. Eyelids should be carefully taped in the closed position and, for surgery in and around the head and neck, protected with padding. The application of 'artificial tears' or chloramphenicol ointment provides additional protection in those patients most at risk. After recent surgery to the eye, or after an eye injury, the use of a plastic eye shield prevents pressure on the eyeball.

## Injury to nerves

Prolonged or permanent injury to nerves is a major cause of postoperative morbidity associated with malpositioning of patients, although as yet unidentified factors in the immediate postoperative period also play a part (Kroll *et al.*, 1990). Nerve damage is often caused by direct pressure and is especially likely in elderly or emaciated patients, or where there are predisposing factors such as a neuropathy. Additional harmful factors such as hypothermia or hypoxia are likely to increase any damage. At particular risk are superficial nerves with a long anatomical course including the ulnar nerve, the radial nerve, the common peroneal nerve and the nerves of the brachial plexus. Brachial plexus injury is caused by placing the arm in an extreme position, particularly if abducted and externally rotated, and this is exacerbated if the neck is extended and flexed in the opposite direction.

In order to prevent nerve injury the patient must be properly positioned and supported, pressure points must be protected and padded, and the arms must not be extended by more than 90° from the body in the sagittal plane.

## *Equipment and the anaesthetized patient*

Monitoring and other equipment in contact with the patient should work satisfactorily and not pose a risk during the anaesthetic. The diathermy plate must be firmly attached to a clean, dry, hairless area. Where the patient might come into contact with bare metal, for example with leg supports attached to the side of the operating table, a protective layer of foam rubber or cotton wool should be inserted between the metal and the patient. After the patient is draped with sterile towels it is often difficult to examine the intravenous access site or alter the placement of the blood pressure cuff and ECG electrodes. These should all be positioned to minimize interference from the surgeon and be checked before surgery commences to ensure that they are working satisfactorily. Where the head and neck are to be covered by towels it is vital to check the integrity and security of the airway and any connections in the breathing circuit before they are lost to view. Endotracheal tubes should be secured in place ensuring that the tube, securing tie, airway and catheter mount do not cause damage by pressure to the mouth and adjacent tissues. The breathing circuit tubing should be supported so as not to drag on the endotracheal tube or to lie across the patient's eyes or face.

## *Maintaining the patient's temperature*

Chapter 6 discusses the impact of environmental temperature on the staff who work in the operating theatre; the point is made that the requirements of the staff are often not the same as those of the patient. Patients lose heat through exposed body surface in a cold environment, and through the use of cold intravenous fluids, cleaning and irrigating solutions. Heat loss is increased during abdominal procedures when the exposed intestines provide a large raw surface area, and is also a particular problem in children who have a relatively large surface area for their mass. Because anaesthesia often vasodilates blood vessels and also abolishes the ability of the patient to increase heat production by shivering, there is little that the patient can do to compensate for any drop in temperature.

It is much easier to prevent heat loss than to warm a patient who has already become cold. In a healthy adult undergoing minor body surface surgery all that is necessary is to maintain a reasonable ambient temperature and to cover with a sheet or blanket all parts of the trunk and limbs that do not require exposure for the operation. For more major procedures, especially those involving intra-abdominal surgery, active steps must be taken to prevent heat loss. These will involve placing the patient on a heating blanket, covering all exposed parts, warming intravenous fluids, as well as all cleaning and irrigating solutions, to 37° Celsius. The patient's core temperature should be monitored and the temperature of the heating blanket must be carefully regulated and observed to ensure that the patient cannot be accidentally burned. Humidifying the inspired gases will also help prevent heat loss and may also decrease the incidence of sore throat in the postoperative period. In small children silver foil may be wrapped around exposed areas, and a reflective blanket performs the same function in adults. For some patients, for example neonates or those with extensive burns, it will be necessary to maintain a high ambient temperature and humidity even if this causes some discomfort to the staff in theatres.

## Handover during a case

Boredom, lack of concentration and fatigue can contribute to anaesthetic-related critical incidents of potential harm to the patient. It is important that the anaesthetist has the opportunity for relaxation and refreshment during a long operation and this will mean handing over to another anaesthetist during the case. It is obvious that in these circumstances there should be a full anaesthetic chart with, in addition to recordings of pulse and blood pressure, a full note of all the drugs and fluids given and accurate timings. Full information and explanation of the conduct of the anaesthetic should be given during the handover to prevent misunderstandings occurring that could endanger the patient. It is important that syringes are clearly labelled with the name and concentration of any drug they contain. The handover also provides an opportunity for a fresh look at an established situation and may in fact identify problems that have been overlooked up to that point by the outgoing anaesthetist (Cooper et al., 1982).

## Blood transfusion

Donor blood is expensive to the National Health Service, potentially hazardous to the patient and never overabundant in supply. It should not be wasted by ordering it when it is not indicated, or by using it when it is not needed. Although there has been some attempt to lay down criteria for cross-matching (Juma *et al.*, 1990), this will clearly depend more on local circumstances than rules devised by others. If the patient is grouped and serum stored in the blood laboratory before operation, cross-matching in most hospitals can be achieved very rapidly when needed. Techniques for limiting blood loss or saving shed blood must also be considered. For certain procedures, such as cardiac surgery, autologous blood donation is attractive providing as it does additional, safe blood and decreasing the need for administration of homologous products (Kay, 1987). The pre-ordering of blood products will depend on local arrangements and requires consultation between the surgeon, anaesthetist and haematologist. It should be remembered that ultimately it will be the anaesthetist who must accept responsibility for any shortfall.

## The anaesthetic technique

The chosen anaesthetic technique can influence the operating conditions during surgery and may alter the risks of complications or even mortality in selected patients. Some considerations for the prevention of postoperative problems are discussed in the section on prophylaxis to prevent complications in Chapter 3.

### General anaesthesia

There is no evidence that individual anaesthetic agents in common use influence mortality in patients in general, although certain agents may be associated with an increased incidence of specific adverse events such as ventricular arrhythmias with halothane and tachycardia with isoflurane (Forrest *et al.*, 1990). Determinants of outcome are multifactorial and depend largely on patient characteristics, and the nature of the procedure. Although the anaesthetic agents as such may not be of prime importance, it is likely that the way they are used will influence outcome. The anaesthetist must therefore be familiar with the techniques and agents used, and administer them in an intelligent, competent and vigilant manner. Some drugs used by the anaesthetist present specific risks to certain individuals. Examples include the dangers of enflurane in an epileptic, or suxamethonium in a patient with recent severe burns or a history of malignant hyperthermia. The anaesthetist must be aware of all the potential dangers and contraindications to these drugs.

*Regional anaesthesia*

Regional anaesthesia carries risks to the patient just as general anaesthesia. The patient must be prepared in the same way, with the same precautions observed and apparatus available. In addition, the patient will be aware of his surroundings because consciousness is not lost, and will require an explanation of the theatre procedure. Care must be taken by the operating theatre staff to preserve a quiet, calm atmosphere, and not to make thoughtless comments that might be heard. Although the patient may be conscious and able to respond to command, full observation and monitoring are still necessary. During a long procedure the patient may wish to listen to music played on a personal stereo system, or talk to a designated member of the operating theatre staff.

Heavy sedation should not be needed during a well-conducted regional anaesthetic, and great care must be exercised when administering central nervous system depressant drugs to these patients. Hypovolaemia is a potent hazard, as effective regional blockade will prevent compensatory vasoconstriction, thus leading to an early fall in blood pressure and a risk of cardiac arrest. Fluid replacement must therefore be meticulous, and many anaesthetists pre-load their patients with intravenous fluid before the local anaesthetic block is undertaken.

All anaesthetists should know the toxic dose of the local anaesthetic to be used and understand that this dose is not solely dependent on weight but can be varied by other factors such as the site of injection, the addition of vasoconstrictors and the concentration of the agent. Agents vary in their toxic effects and special care should be taken when using bupivacaine as its cardiotoxic properties may make resuscitation difficult after an overdose.

## Awareness under anaesthesia

A recent study in anaesthetized nonobstetric patients reported an incidence of awareness with recall of 0.2%, and of dreaming under anaesthesia of 0.9% (Liu *et al.*, 1991). Review of previous studies suggests that the incidence has decreased over the last 30 years. There is a spectrum of awareness from full recall and pain, through awareness but no pain, experience of unpleasant dreams and amnesic wakefulness, finally to the ability to induce post-anaesthetic suggestions (Griffiths and Jones, 1990). A patient who has been aware under an anaesthetic may develop a subsequent neurosis, and this may be made worse if it is suggested that the experience was imaginary. If such an untoward event is treated by all concerned with sympathetic understanding and a full explanation given, it may avoid some claims for medical negligence. Awareness usually arises from a faulty anaesthetic technique, particularly with a paralysed patient, although less commonly there may be equipment malfunction. Unfortunately there is as yet no simple and reliable monitor of depth of anaesthesia. Successful defence against complaints of awareness can only be made if there is a comprehensive anaesthetic record which details the dose, concentrations and timings of all drugs as well as frequent recordings of vital signs (Aitkenhead, 1990).

## References

Aitkenhead, A. R. (1990) Awareness during anaesthesia: what should the patient be told? *Anaesthesia*, **45**, 351–352

Allen, E. V. (1929) Thromboangitis obliterans. Method of diagnosing chronic occlusive arterial lesions distal to the wrist with illustrative cases. *American Journal of Medical Science*, **178**, 237–244

Allison, A. and McCrory, J. (1990) Tracheal placement of a gum elastic bougie using the laryngeal mask airway. *Anaesthesia*, **45**, 419–420

Association of Anaesthetists of Great Britain and Ireland (1990) *Checklist for Anaesthetic Machines*, London

Bogod, D. G. (1990) General anaesthesia in the presence of a spouse. *Anaesthesia*, **45**, 422–423

Boyce, J. R. and Peters, G. L. (1989) Vessel dilator cricothyrotomy for transtracheal jet ventilation. *Canadian Journal of Anaesthesia*, **36**, 350–353

Calder, I., Ordman, A. J., Jackowski, A. and Crockard, H. A. (1990) The Brain laryngeal mask airway; an alternative to emergency tracheal intubation. *Anaesthesia*, **45**, 137–139

Caplan, R. A., Posner, K. L., Ward, R. J. and Cheney, F. W. (1990) Adverse respiratory events in anesthesia: a closed claims analysis. *Anesthesiology*, **72**, 828–833

Cooper, J. B., Long, C. D., Newbower, R. S. and Philip, J. H. (1982) Critical incidents associated with intraoperative exchanges of anesthesia personnel. *Anesthesiology*, **56**, 456–461

Cooper, J. B., Newbower, R. S. and Kitz, R. J. (1984) An analysis of major errors and equipment failures in anesthesia management: consideration for prevention and detection. *Anesthesiology*, **60**, 34–42

Crosby, W. M. (1988) Checking the anaesthetic machine, drugs, and monitoring devices. *Anaesthesia and Intensive Care*, **16**, 32–35

Forrest, J. B., Cahalan, M. K., Rehder, K., Goldsmith, C. H., Levy, W. J., Strunin, L., Bota, W., Boucek, C. D., Cucchiara, R. F., Dhamee, S., Domino, K. B., Dudman, A. J., Hamilton, W. K., Kampine, J., Kotrly, K. J., Maltby, J. R., Mazloomdoost, M., Mackenzie, R. A., Melnick, B. M., Motoyama, E., Muir, J. J. and Munshi, C. (1990) Multicenter study of general anesthesia. II. Results. *Anesthesiology*, **72**, 262–268

Gould, M. J. (1989) Preoxygenation. *British Journal of Anaesthesia*, **62**, 241–242

Griffiths, D. and Jones, J. G. (1990) Awareness and memory in anaesthetized patients. *British Journal of Anaesthesia*, **65**, 603–606

Hannallah, R. S. and Rosales, J. K. (1983) Experience with parents' presence during anaesthesia induction in children. *Canadian Anaesthetists' Society Journal*, **30**, 286–289

Heath, M. L. and Allagain, J. (1990) The Brain laryngeal mask airway as an aid to intubation. *British Journal of Anaesthesia*, **64**, 382p–383p.

Hecker, J. F. (1989) Failure of intravenous infusions from extravasation and phlebitis. *Anaesthesia and Intensive Care*, **17**, 433–439

Juma, T., Baraka, A., Abu-Lisan, M. and Asfar, S. K. (1990) Blood ordering for elective surgery: time for a change. *Journal of the Royal Society of Medicine*, **83**, 368–370

Kaplan, J. A. (1979) Hemodynamic monitoring. In *Cardiac Anesthesia* (Ed. Kaplan, J. A.), Grune and Stratton, New York, pp. 71–115

Kay, L. A. (1987) The need for autologous blood transfusion. *British Medical Journal*, **1**, 137–138

Kroll, D. A., Caplan, R. A., Posner, K., Ward, R. J. and Cheney, F. W. (1990) Nerve injury associated with anesthesia. *Anesthesiology*, **73**, 202–207

Kumar, V., Barcellos, W. A., Mehta, M. P. and Carter, J. G. (1988) An analysis of critical incidents in a teaching department for quality assurance. A survey of mishaps during anaesthesia. *Anaesthesia*, **43**, 879–883

Lewis, G. B. H. and Hecker, J. F. (1985) Infusion thrombophlebitis. *British Journal of Anaesthesia*, **57**, 220–233

Liu, W. H. D., Thorp, T. A. S., Graham, S. G. and Aitkenhead, A. R. (1991) Incidence of awareness with recall during general anaesthesia. *Anaesthesia*, **46**, 435–437

Mallampati, R. S., Gatt, S. P., Guginao, L. D., Desai, S. P., Waraksa, B., Freiberger, D. and Liu, P. L. (1985) A clinical sign to predict difficult tracheal intubation: a prospective study. *Canadian Anaesthetists' Society Journal*, **32**, 429–434

Safar, P. and Pennickx, J. (1967) Cricothyroid membrane puncture with a special cannula. *Anesthesiology*, **28**, 943–948

Samsoon, G. L. T. and Young, J. R. B. (1987) Difficult tracheal intubation: a retrospective study. *Anaesthesia*, **42**, 487–490

Schofield, N. McC. and White, J. B. (1989) Interrelations among children, parents, premedication, and anaesthetists in paediatric day stay surgery. *British Medical Journal*, **299**, 1371–1375

Slogoff, S., Keats, A. S. and Arlund, C. (1983) On the safety of radial artery cannulation. *Anesthesiology*, **59**, 42–47

Tordoff, S. G. and Sweeney, B. P. (1990) Intravenous cannulae colour coding; a perennial source of confusion. *Anaesthesia*, **45**, 399–400

Tunstall, M. E. (1976) Failed intubation drill. *Anaesthesia*, **31**, 850

Vaughan, R. S. (1989) Airways revisited (Editorial). *British Journal of Anaesthesia*, **62**, 1–3

# 5

# Monitoring and recording

It is still true to say that the continuous presence of an expert anaesthetist during the course of an operation, provided that individual is alert and exercising his or her powers of observation, is the first essential for adequate intraoperative monitoring of an anaesthetized patient. The use of simple monitoring apparatus forms a valuable addition to clinical observation, and indeed is now thought to be essential in most developed countries. There are many individuals in the professional bodies of anaesthetists throughout the world who believe the introduction of obligatory minimum standards of monitoring will further enhance safety and prevent some of the anaesthetic mishaps leading to permanent sequelae such as death or brain damage. There is evidence in the literature to support this view. In some countries this feeling is so strong that the use of certain monitors has been made compulsory by law. Thus, in New York State, minimal monitoring is compulsory for any patient given an anaesthetic via an endothracheal tube. The corollary of this is that all practising anaesthetists must be fully conversant with the monitoring system employed, be able to react correctly to the readings displayed and be familiar with the shortcomings of the apparatus. It is also essential that all compulsory monitors are fitted with alarms.

In some parts of the world, when fit patients undergo routine minor procedures the attention of the anaesthetist, unsupplemented by monitoring devices, still suffices, provided observation is made at all times of the patient's respiratory pattern, chest movements and skin colour, and the attendant palpates a peripheral pulse and extrapolates from this the adequacy of the cardiac output. It is highly unlikely that all minor operations are observed conscientiously and continuously in this way. Furthermore, as the defence organizations and insurance companies are aware, many tragedies occur because of human error or lack of knowledge, leading to misinterpretation of the signs observed. Attention wanders from the observation of the patient and interpretation of the data is not uniform. If the projected operation is more complex, or if the patient is less fit, the clinical observation of the patient may not give sufficient information early enough to ensure the patient's wellbeing. For these reasons it has become essential to use monitoring apparatus routinely on anaesthetized patients. Thus the need for complex perioperative monitoring systems has been built up, despite the fact that until some 30 years ago even major procedures were conducted with only clinical observation of the patient supplemented by intermittent blood pressure recordings by means of a cuff and a brachial stethoscope, and a continuously running electrocardiogram (ECG). Similarly, it is now acknowledged that the period of close observation needed for patient safety starts before induction and extends after the operation until full recovery is secure.

It remains, therefore, that many anaesthetics for uncomplicated procedures lasting less than 30 minutes in an ASA I or II patient are given by a mask with simple clinical monitoring only. But, even in these circumstances the addition of basic monitoring apparatus, for example a pulse oximeter, must enhance the safety without detracting from the skill and ability of the anaesthetist. As the complexity of events increases the simple methods become less effective and more elaborate monitoring is required, but it is essential that those who use this equipment are familiar with it and the limitations of the apparatus and the results are clearly understood.

## Clinical monitoring

The most widely available monitoring techniques are the ECG and non-invasive blood pressure measurement (NIBP). Their use should not be neglected, but they are primarily of value for the control of the actual anaesthetic process, and especially the quantity and type of drugs given; they are of little value for the early detection of disaster (Weingarten, 1986). This is a further reason for the need to employ more sophisticated and appropriate apparatus, if patients are to be protected from the consequences of tragic mishaps.

## Monitoring apparatus

It is now necessary to identify the useful and practical means of monitoring a patient from the multitude of pieces of apparatus available. The authors have no intention of advocating a particular type of apparatus, or that of a particular manufacturer. In the succeeding pages reference will only be made to those types of monitor which are easily applied to a patient by a competent individual working in the environment of a normal district general hospital in the United

**Table 5.1   Monitorising: functions and apparatus**

1. Monitoring the gas supply
    Oxygen supply failure alarm
    Inspired oxygen analyser
    High pressure alarm
    Disconnection alarm
    Expired respiratory volume
    End-tidal $CO_2$
    Expired volatile agent

2. Monitoring the patient
    Correct tube placement
        See passage through cords
        Capnograph (ETCO$_2$)
        Aspiration syringe
        Stethoscope
    Heart rate and rhythm
        Palpation
        Electrocardiogram (ECG)
        Pulsemeter
        Pulse oximeter
        Stethoscope
    Oxygen saturation
        Pulse oximeter
    Respiratory rate depth
        Observation
        Respirometer
        Capnograph (ETCO$_2$)
    Blood pressure
        Noninvasive (NIBP)
        Invasive (IBP)
    Right atrial pressure
        Central venous catheter (CVP)
    Pulmonary capillary wedge pressure
        Pulmonary artery catheter
    Cardiac output
        Pulmonary artery catheter and thermodilution
    Blood loss
        Swab weigh
        Colorimetric
        Resistivity
    Blood gases
        Arterial sample
    Body temperature
        Oesophageal or rectal probe
    Depth of anaesthesia
        Clinical
        Electroencephalogram (EEG)
        Evoked potentials
        Oesophageal contractility
        Frontalis muscle response
    Neuromuscular blockade
        Perhpheral nerve stimulator
    Urine output
        Volume from catheter

Kingdom. If the addition of complicated and ill understood apparatus merely distracts the observer from proper clinical observation, the patient is put at risk with no enhancement of the safety of the anaesthetic. The monitors available will be discussed under two headings, those monitoring the delivery of gases and apparatus function, and those monitoring the patient.

It is perhaps unfortunate that there is little that can be done to monitor the performance of the anaesthetist, for the majority of errors are due to human failing. Sykes suggests that a degree of self-monitoring could be induced by developing set routines in anaesthetic practice (Sykes, 1987). Many disastrous accidents can be avoided by close clinical observation of the patient and conscious attention to the gas delivery system. Reviewing the notes of such cases does frequently seem to reveal a failure in these simple routines.

It should not be necessary to state that the anaesthetist's eyes, ears and hands should be continuously employed in assessing and recording the patient's condition, from the moment before induction until the patient is handed over to the care of a skilled recovery ward nurse. The information gained in this way by the anaesthetist should be supplemented by the correct monitoring apparatus. Table 5.1 shows the functions to be monitored and the possible method and apparatus that could be used for this purpose. The advantages and disadvantages of each will be discussed.

## Monitoring the gas supply

The presence of an anaesthetist constantly checking the anaesthetic machine and circuits by observation and by examination can provide a measure of protection against equipment failure or disconnection. But however attentive the individual, this cannot be as efficient as the correct alarms, activated and in circuit. Nowhere is this more important than in ensuring an adequate oxygen supply, because direct measurement is the only sure way to assess that oxygen in the set percentage is being delivered at all times during an anaesthetic (Brahams, 1989). When the absence of such a device leads to a dead or brain damaged patient, the cost of the apparatus is small compared with the cost in real terms for the compensation of a damaged patient and in personal terms for the distress of relatives.

### Oxygen supply failure alarms

Oxygen failure alarms are clearly critical when the patient is dependent upon supplies from a cylinder, as the gas is limited in quantity and the duration of the supply is ill-defined. The use of pipeline gases in most hospitals has made absolute failure of supply to the machine rare. However, all machines, whether supplied by cylinder or pipeline, should incorporate an oxygen failure device which is activated when the pressure on the delivery side is reduced. Ideally these should at the same time progressively reduce or cut off the supply of nitrous oxide. A distinctive audible alarm is essential to warn the anaesthetist and others present in the operating theatre (Memorandum, 1977).

### Inspired oxygen analyser

Since most modern hospitals rely on pipeline supplies it is more likely that the patient would be deprived of oxygen because of a fault in the delivery system rather than a failure of supply. Cases where there has been contamination of the pipeline supply and instances of pipeline misconnections have been reported, but these are rare because of the detailed regulations that are now imposed before newly commissioned pipelines can be used (Health Technical Memorandum, 1972). It is therefore necessary to have an oxygen failure alarm in the patient's gas system as near to the patient as possible, certainly beyond the common gas outflow from the machine. This may be a separate unit or incorporated in an end-tidal carbon dioxide analyser. If this apparatus is inserted into the inspiratory limb of the circuit there is a danger that it may not detect a low volume in the total gas flow. In this situation, even when the percentage of oxygen in the mixture is satisfactory, hypoxia may result. If the device is placed in the expiratory limb of the circuit this danger does not arise, for the percentage of oxygen in the expired gases would be low in the circumstances mentioned and the alarm would be activated. For the former site a lower limit of 25% is recommended for most patients, but for the latter the lower level of 21% is required. An upper limit of about 40% may be used in either place to detect nitrous oxide failure. These alarms are now firmly recommended by the manufacturers of anaesthetic machines, and are required to comply with the recommendations of the checklist for use with anaesthetic machines issued by the Association of Anaesthetists of Great Britain and Ireland (see also Chapter 4).

### High pressure alarm

Most anaesthetic machines and ventilators have a relief valve which vents the circuit to the atmosphere once a preset pressure has been exceeded. The value set by the manufacturers is usually much higher than that desirable for full protection of the lungs in all patients, especially the frail. Most ventilator disconnection alarms allow a high pressure limit to be set, above which the apparatus will alarm, and this should be set to protect the patient from excess pressure in the circuit and to warn of obstruction in the connecting tubing. To be fully effective the alarms must be set for each patient by the anaesthetist, and may need adjustment during a procedure (Pryn and Crosse, 1989).

## Disconnection alarms

Disconnection alarms give an audible warning when a certain pressure is not reached within the circuit in a given period of time, thus detecting the failure of a ventilator to cycle effectively. The assumption is that the pressure rises from a low or zero level to a higher pressure during each respiratory cycle. The time factor built into the alarm is constant, between 15 and 20 seconds, for the rate of respiration would normally be above 3 or 4 min, but the low pressure which acts as the threshold for the warning device can often be preset by the anaesthetist. The preferred level set is usually around 7 $cmH_2O$. It is important not to set a level that is too low as there is danger that the pressure may never fall back below this at any time during the cycle. This is because of the resistance to flow in the circuit, which may maintain the pressure above the preset lower limit so that the alarm will never work (Pryn and Crosse, 1989). The resistance of the circuit may be increased by the addition of capnograph cuvettes and heat and moisture exchangers. A further example of a dangerous situation due to the resistance of the circuit not falling below the 'alarm' level is when there is a disconnection at the endotracheal tube connector, usually the narrowest part of the patient circuit. The small diameter constitutes a resistance to flow, thus allowing the pressure to remain above the alarm level set, despite the complete disconnection of the circuit to the patient. This could be the explanation for the failure of a disconnection alarm leading to severe brain damage and death which resulted in an anaesthetist being convicted of manslaughter at the Old Bailey in January 1990.

## Expired respiratory volume

Ideally the difference between the inspired and expired gas volume should be used to detect significant leaks in the patient circuit. To construct an alarm from such information would require an electronic integrator and therefore be costly. The measurement is not essential in patients who are breathing spontaneously or being ventilated by hand, but some confirmation of the integrity of the circuit and the gas in it is required during intermittent positive pressure ventilation (IPPV) with a machine. Estimating the expired gas volume at the expiratory port of a minute volume divider ventilator will allow the anaesthetist to make a comparison with the theoretical inspired minute volume set by the rotameters and assist in detecting leaks from the circuit. The Wright respirometer is a small anenometer which can carry out this function, although it is somewhat susceptible to condensation of the expired water vapour.

*End-tidal carbon dioxide*

The end-tidal carbon dioxide level is a guide to the adequacy of respiration and ventilation. It is possible to achieve low levels with hyperventilation by machine. The sample for this purpose must be taken from near the endotracheal tube. A peak carbon dioxide level would be sufficient for this, but this monitor can also subserve other functions if inspired and end-tidal expired carbon dioxide are measured. This function is probably more important in the context of patient monitoring and will be considered later. The capnograph also has a more specific function in the detection of air embolism, which is indicated by a sudden fall in the level of the end-tidal carbon dioxide.

*Expired volatile anaesthetic agent*

The percentage of expired volatile agent can be measured by an infra-red absorption device (Ilsley *et al.*, 1986) or by mass spectrometry. The former should be placed near the patient but out of the breathing circuit directly, and is useful to make sure the correct agent is delivered, and also for detecting overdosage (due, for example, to a fault in the vaporizer calibration) and low dosage (due, for example, to the vaporizer being empty or oxygen bypass remaining on) and thus preventing awareness. The monitor can also be used to check the accuracy of the vaporizers themselves, although most anaesthetists rely implicitly on the inherent accuracy of adequately serviced apparatus for use with volatile agents.

## Monitoring the patient

Most of the activities for monitoring the patient can be carried out clinically. However, additional monitoring provides continuity, quantifies clinical findings and gives information which is either not available or not available early enough for patient safety. Although the fitting of alarms, which can be adjusted by the anaesthetist for each patient, is useful, the instrument should be capable of continuing its monitoring function even when the alarm is actuated. The construction of some monitors does not allow this, and manufacturers should modify those that do not to provide this continuous monitoring. It is desirable that the data from these instruments should be displayed for easy visibility at a distance, and this information should ideally be recorded by the machine with real time marked. The information thus captured should be printed out to form a record of the anaesthetic for the patient's notes, and such hard copy should always be preserved.

In this section mention will be made of the simple clinical methods for monitoring each function before discussing the apparatus that can be used to improve the information obtained.

*Correct placement of the endotracheal tube*

This may be done clinically by observing the movements of the chest wall and by auscultating the chest and, in cases where there is doubt, also listening over the stomach. The movement of the chest wall must be closely observed, noting any asymmetry. There is ample evidence both in the world literature and the records of the Defence Societies to show that this method is fallible and this fallibility can lead to failure to detect an oesophageal intubation until severe hypoxia ensues. Thus, in the case of a difficult intubation, where it has proved impossible to see the endotracheal tube pass through the vocal cords, it is essential to institute further checks, including, as previously mentioned, auscultation over the upper abdomen as well as the lung fields (Andersen and Hald, 1989). It should not be necessary to state that if a patient appears to be cyanosed when an endotracheal tube is in place and proper ventilation instituted, then serious doubt must be thrown on the placement of the tube. The position must be carefully checked as the first priority, and if there is any doubt that it is in the trachea it must be removed and oxygen administered by a mask. Since fit patients frequently react to hypoxia by a progressive bradycardia following a brief tachycardia which is often not observed, the correct placement of the endotracheal tube should be confirmed immediately if this alteration in rate is seen.

Oesophageal intubation can be simply detected by connecting a large 50 ml syringe to the tube with a suitable connector and aspirating. No gas is obtained if the tube is in the oesophagus, while in correct intubation of the trachea, free entry of air into the syringe is easily obtained (Wee, 1988).

Absolute confirmation that the endotracheal tube is indeed in the trachea can be given by an end-tidal carbon dioxide analyser. This will show a free swing from zero to an upper level with a correctly placed tube and this swing coincides with the respiration in both spontaneous and artificial ventilation. With the tube in the oesophagus no swing will be detected, the level remaining low or on zero. The apparatus will show disconnections or ventilator failure because there will be no difference in inspired and expired carbon dioxide, the so-called 'apnoea alarm' situation. The alarm is important, but it is essential at this time that the monitoring function should not be overridden by the alarm, as happens with much current apparatus. The capnograph will not detect the intubation of only one lung or the obstruction of one bronchus by the balloon, and a high index of suspicion, leading to observation of the chest movements and auscultation, is needed to detect this at an early stage. A low oxygen saturation is also a pointer to this problem. Most capnographs incorporate an expired oxygen meter and a respiratory rate meter.

*Heart rate and rhythm*

This may again be assessed clinically, either with a stethoscope or by palpation, or continuously throughout an operation by means of a monaural oesophageal stethoscope. These can be obtained with a radio connection, enabling the anaesthetist to move freely around the operating theatre. This stethoscope has the advantage of monitoring breath sounds as well as the heart sounds, but it is difficult to maintain this method continuously throughout a long anaesthetic, and at times the concentration of the anaesthetist may lapse.

Traditionally an ECG displayed on an oscilloscope has been used to detect variations and abnormalities of heart rate and rhythm, and this monitor has been in use for many years and is still the one most consistently employed during anaesthesia. It is the only monitor that can identify that exact nature of a dysrhythmia for it not only demonstrates at a glance the heart rate and rhythm, but if printed out or 'frozen' on a screen, can be used for more detailed diagnosis. A good trace using the appropriate leads will also show ST segment changes indicating possible ischaemia. The chief fault of the apparatus is that there is no indication in the trace of the adequacy of peripheral circulation, and the trace may appear relatively normal, at least in the short term, in patients with gross circulatory failure to the brain. Indeed it is the common experience of the Defence Societies that in cases of death or brain damage due to oxygen lack during anaesthesia, the first indication of severe hypoxia was a bradycardia observed by the anaesthetist on an ECG screen. Furthermore, this was often treated in the first instance with an anticholinergic drug such as atropine. This is a classic example of human error in anaesthetic mishaps and, although not directly attributable to the method of monitoring, it can be eliminated by the use of other apparatus.

A modified lead 5 or CM5 is the best compromise if only a single lead of the ECG is employed, as it is the lead that will show the highest percentage of dysrhythmias, but at the same time give most evidence of myocardial ischaemia (Foëx and Prys-Roberts, 1974). For this trace the right arm electrode of lead 1 is placed over the sternum (central manubrium, hence CM), the left arm electrode over the left fifth intercostal space (hence 5) in the anterior axillary line, and the indifferent electrode on the left shoulder.

The simple pulsemeter also shows heart rate and can demonstrate some irregularity of rhythm. This device often has an audible signal. Some models may give some indication of cardiac output volume and if used in conjunction with a manometer cuff on the same arm can be used for intraoperative blood pressure measurement. They become unreliable when there is patient (or surgical) movement and if there is hypovolaemia and therefore poor peripheral perfusion.

The pulse oximeter can also be used to display pulse rate and an irregularity in the heart rhythm, in addition to the oxygen saturation. The rate is usually shown digitally, but the rhythm has to be deduced from the display of successive pulse beats. This is easy if the display is in the form of a pulse curve, but less so when it is a repeated blip. Unlike the ECG, this trace clearly has little diagnostic value. Digital displays on most pieces of apparatus are clear and discernible from across an operating theatre. The further uses of this apparatus are discussed below.

## Oxygen saturation

Oxygen saturation is displayed digitally on a pulse oximeter. Various probes are designed to be placed on a finger, toe, ear or nasal septum. A low saturation alarm can be set by the anaesthetist, and this makes the equipment very useful during induction of anaesthesia and in the recovery area. The authors believe that it is useful in all patients in the recovery room, but it should be mandatory to use this apparatus during the early period of recovery in non-white patients, especially children. These last are especially vulnerable to unobserved hypoxaemia in this situation.

The pulse oximeter is a late measure of the integrity of both the cardiovascular and respiratory systems, and also of the correct delivery of oxygen from the anaesthetic machine. Although it is highly accurate, to around 1%, if the lower alarm limit is set at a low level the patient will require quick and positive action from the anaesthetist to prevent the onset of severe hypoxia and possible subsequent damage. It is unreliable in hypotensive, hypothermic or intensely vasoconstricted patients, or in the presence of high levels of carboxyhaemoglobin. The user must have available various types of probes, to facilitate its use in all surgical procedures and when peripheral perfusion varies. It functions satisfactorily in the presence of cyanosis (Taylor and Whitwam, 1986).

## Respiratory rate and depth

During spontaneous ventilation the rate and depth of respiration may be assessed by observing the motion of the patient's chest and the 'reservoir bag'. With machine ventilation the depth of respiration is usually set by the anaesthetist's adjustment of the tidal volume and the chest can be observed for the rate if there is no automatic dial reading provided.

Many ventilators show the rate of respiration and this is also often found on end-tidal carbon dioxide monitors. The respiratory tidal volume may be measured by an anemometer, such as the Wright. As has already been discussed in the section on monitoring of the gas supply, this is a useful piece of equipment on a ventilator to compare the expected tidal volume with that actually coming from the patient. This will enable early detection of a leak in the circuit and prevent the possibility of hypoxia.

*Arterial blood pressure*

Clinically the blood pressure can be measured in the traditional way, listening for the Koratkoff sounds with a stethoscope at the brachial artery and measuring the cuff pressure with an aneroid dial or a mercury column. The end point can also be taken by palpating the pulse, by loss of the pulse as shown by a pulse oximeter, pulsemeter or doppler probe, or by the oscillation of the pointer of an oscillo-tonometer or similar device. These indirect measurements have a wide variability in both magnitude and direction of error and this is made worse by hypovolaemia and poor peripheral perfusion (Runciman, Rutten and Ilsley, 1981). Estimations are often not completed at the prescribed times during an anaesthetic, which should be at 5 minute intervals with greater frequency at critical times. It is therefore essential to have automatic apparatus that takes pressures at preset intervals, and these should ideally have a full recording capability with real time printout. When considering the trend of such a recording it should be remembered that there can be an in-built error in these readings. The interval between automatic readings should not be routinely set at less than 5 minutes, for shorter intervals have caused oedema and swelling of the arm, as venous engorgement persists between readings.

Compared to the indirect methods, a direct arterial pressure reading is more accurate, continuous and usually more reliable, but is not without undesirable sequelae in some patients due to local damage to the artery from the indwelling cannula. In addition, there is a continuous danger of air embolism and haemorrhage from the puncture site while the cannula is in place. The apparatus should display the pressure digitally and show the pulse wave, and it is convenient if a recording can be made during anaesthesia. Access to the circulation is gained by means of a cannula in a peripheral artery, usually the radial of the non-dominant side. It would be ideal if the collateral flow in the vessels to the fingers could be reliably tested, although in major operations, even if there were some doubt of the integrity of this blood flow, the requirement for continuous arterial pressure display may be paramount. Unfortunately, simple tests of collateral blood flow to the hand and digits are of little value in predicting problems. Loss of distal blood supply, with consequent amputation of part or all of some digits, is rare, but the possibility should always be considered when contemplating invasive arterial monitoring. The danger to peripheral flow is not completely eliminated by the use of bigger vessels, such as the brachial or the femoral artery.

A simple aneroid manometer can be used to give a mean pressure from an indwelling cannula, but more sophisticated apparatus is desirable. By using a transducer and a monitor the pulse wave can be demonstrated and both the systolic/diastolic or the mean pressure shown. The apparatus must be properly calibrated before use and ideally should have a recorder to provide a permanent record when required. Some attention must be paid to the damping in the system, as most over-read systolic and under-read diastolic pressures. The system must be sufficiently sensitive to produce the peaks and troughs of the wave form.

## Right atrial pressure

Precise diagnosis of the perioperative cause of hypotension, and therefore the management of fluid balance, can be difficult in the old and sick, when rapid alterations in fluid load may be dangerous. To guide fluid therapy in these cases it is now accepted that the inherent complications of the use of central venous or pulmonary artery catheters are outweighed by the advantages gained from the information they supply during treatment. The measurements that require the use of long catheters include right atrial pressure, pulmonary capillary wedge pressure and cardiac output.

Right atrial pressure is often referred to as central venous pressure. It requires the insertion of a long catheter into a central vein, either from the brachial vein in the arm, the internal jugular vein in the neck, the femoral vein in the groin or via the subclavian vein. This is connected to either a fluid column or a pressure transducer. The former is simple to set up and provides an accurate mean pressure, but is cumbersome and requires constant adjustment, while the latter allows a display of the wave form, shows the effect of ventilation on the pressure and can provide a recording of the actual pressures, although it is subject to all the usual drawbacks of such apparatus. The fluid column method is subject to greater error if IPPV is employed with a large respiratory excursion, but whatever method of measurement is employed, an end-expiratory value should be the one recorded (Runciman, Rutten and Ilsley, 1981).

## Pulmonary capillary wedge pressure

In 1970 Swan and Ganz and colleagues introduced a multilumened, polyvinyl catheter that could be passed into the pulmonary artery by flotation without the need for X-ray control. Over the next few years this device was developed for many monitoring and therapeutic purposes. A device of this type can be used to measure the pressure in the pulmonary artery and also the pressure of the pulmonary capillary bed, hence providing an estimate of the pressure of the left atrium. Modifications of this catheter can also give a mixed venous sample for haemoglobin saturation and the right ventricular ejection fraction, as well as providing the means to pace the left ventricle electrically. Both pressures are measured from the distal lumen, the former when there is free flow into the lungs around the catheter and the latter by isolating the tip from the pressure of the right ventricle by wedging the catheter by means of a balloon, or by actually inserting the catheter far enough to exclude the pressure.

The most commonly employed catheter in adults is a 7 French gauge Swan–Ganz with four channels. The distal end of the catheter is open to one lumen, another is used to inflate a small balloon just behind the tip, there is an opening about 15 cm from the catheter tip which should open into the right atrium on correct placement and the last lumen carries the wires for a thermistor situated 4 cm from the catheter tip. The catheter can measure pulmonary artery pressure and pulmonary capillary wedge pressure, properly called the pulmonary artery occlusion pressure, from the distal aperture, and by injecting cold solution into the atrial lumen and measuring the distal temperature with the thermistor the cardiac output from a thermodilution curve can be derived. The balloon assists flotation through the chambers of the heart, helps to protect the endothelial surfaces of the heart during passage of the catheter, and is used to occlude the pulmonary flow past the tip when measuring pulmonary capillary wedge pressure. Therapeutic injections of drugs or fluids can also be given into the right atrium via the atrial lumen.

The insertion of these catheters is not easy and should only be carried out by properly trained staff. The pressures may be useful during anaesthesia, but they can be of vital importance during the immediate postoperative period in sick patients. These include those with a low cardiac output, or with pulmonary oedema, and in patients to be treated with large quantities of intravenous fluid. Once inserted, the catheter can provide a continuous trace of the pulmonary capillary bed at the end of expiration. This pressure is usually a good estimate of the pressure in the left atrium, and provides a guide to fluid management. As with many pressure measurements, trends are more important than single values.

*Cardiac output*

This can be determined, using a thermodilution technique, by injecting a cold solution into the atrial lumen of a Swan–Ganz catheter. The thermistor at the tip provides the input for the computer which assesses flow from the alteration in temperature over time and hence calculates the cardiac output. The accuracy is comparable with a formal dye-dilution technique, provided the catheter is correctly placed and the solution, which must be injected rapidly, is at around 0 degrees centigrade when administered. Modern cardiac output computers will also measure the temperature of the injectate as well as that of the catheter tip, and thus increase the accuracy of the measurement. The accuracy is sufficient for clinical purposes. It is usual to average three measurements within the same phase of respiration.

Cardiac output can also be measured in the clinical setting by doppler, either by the transoesophageal or suprasternal route. This method will reflect changes in output, but an estimate or a measurement of the aortic root diameter is needed for absolute values to be estimated. Echocardiography is more complex, and at present probably only suitable for research purposes during the intraoperative period. Impedance techniques provide a possible means of noninvasive measurement of cardiac output, although the reliability of this method has still to be demonstrated in clinical practice.

## Surgical blood loss

The measurement of blood loss should be instituted for major procedures and those expected to lead to an appreciable loss. The simple method of estimating the loss is to use only dry swabs and towels, unless wetted from a known measured source of saline, which is also used if wound irrigation is required. The blood loss can then be found by weighing the swabs, subtracting the weight of the dry swabs used and adding the weight of the suctioned fluid and from this total deducting the weight of the measured saline used. The result must be the added weight of the blood actually lost by the patient. To ensure accuracy all blood lost should be included as far as possible in the calculation, and it must be kept up to date throughout the procedure, to ensure little loss by evaporation of water from the swabs. This is particularly important when employing the method in children. The method consistently underestimates the actual blood loss, and most anaesthetists would add up to one-third to the measured volume to provide a better estimate. Water and blood have the same weight for the purposes of this calculation.

More complicated methods of estimating blood loss have been described using colorimetry or resistivity to assess the concentration of haemoglobin or electrolytes respectively in a large volume of fluid. These techniques are useful in operations such as transurethral resection of the prostate or bladder tumour, and in the removal of the endometrium by endoscopic means. They may be applicable when great accuracy is desired for clinical or research purposes, especially when large losses are anticipated.

However accurate the determination of blood loss is thought to be, and hence the adequacy of the blood replacement, it is important that the haemoglobin levels should be measured at appropriate intervals in the postoperative period.

### Measurement of blood gases

The facility to measure the blood gases from an arterial sample should be available in all situations where anaesthetics are administered except for the most trivial cases. Arterial blood gas analysis provides a measure of the adequacy of ventilation, and more specifically the efficiency of oxygenation and carbon dioxide removal. The pH and the bicarbonate reflect the patient's acid–base status, and allow the anaesthetist to assess whether the pH alterations are due to metabolic or respiratory causes.

### Body temperature

This is a simple measurement to make, but is not widely used in routine anaesthesia in the United Kingdom. It is more strongly advocated in the United States, and should receive more emphasis elsewhere for it is a safe, noninvasive measurement easily identifying changes from normal body temperature. The temperature required is that of the body core and can most usefully be obtained by using an oesophageal or rectal probe. The method can detect falls of temperature that may occur with large volume transfusions, as well as in prolonged operations, especially those in which large body cavities are opened, as in abdominal surgery. Children are most at risk because they have a large body surface area, from which heat is lost, relative to adults, and their metabolic needs are higher. In adults temperature falls may lead to excessive shivering in the recovery period, and this can be harmful in the frail and the elderly. It will also give warning of temperature rises, although in malignant hyperpyrexia the sudden rise in expired carbon dioxide levels is an earlier warning, and this itself may be preceded by tachycardia and hyperventilation.

### Depth of anaesthesia

The fact that the level of anaesthesia is difficult to assess at the present time is self-evident from the reported cases of awareness under general anaesthesia reaching the courts of law in pursuit of damages. In 1970, Brice, Hetherington and Utting defined awareness as 'the ability to recall, with or without prompting, events which occurred during the period at which it was thought that the patient was fully unconscious'. The majority of cases of awareness are due to failure of the anaesthetist to administer sufficient anaesthetic drugs when supervising patients who are paralysed (70%), or failure to check the apparatus before use (20%), with few due to technical circuit failure and other causes

(Hargrove, 1987). It is probably true that the incidence of awareness is directly related to the depth of anaesthesia in a given procedure, and this conflicts somewhat with the perceived benefits of administering a 'light' anaesthetic during an operation. Thus, it is desirable to be able to evaluate the exact depth of each anaesthetic.

The need to determine the depth of anaesthesia accurately is crucial when a patient has received a muscle relaxant, for these drugs abolish reactive movements during surgery, and therefore reliance has to be placed on other signs. Clinical assessment is easy to perform and is probably the best indicator available at the present time, although unfortunately none of the signs are absolutely reliable. The most valuable signs are those that reveal stimulation of the sympathetic system, including systolic arterial pressure, heart rate, lacrimation and sweating. Although attempts have been made to devise scoring systems which accurately predict the exact depth of anaesthesia from these and other signs, they have not been found to be useful, partly because there are no values of these clinical signs that can accurately predict awareness, but also many of the component signs are directly affected by the agents given in the normal course of the anaesthetic. For example, atropine and other vagolytic drugs increase heart rate, beta-blockers prevent tachycardia and increases in blood pressure, and sweating is also affected by the ambient temperature. They would also be affected by local and regional analgesia.

It would seem to be logical that the study of an electroencephalogram (EEG) would provide information about the depth of anaesthesia. This hope has not been realized because of the extreme complexity of the waveform and hence the difficulty in interpretation. This has led to the rejection of the diagnostic EEG machine for the purpose, although several attempts have been made to process the signal to produce a simpler trace and thus a more obvious measure of depth of anaesthesia. The cerebral function monitor (CFM) records an integrated EEG trace, which shows alterations in overall amplitude in response to the changes in depth of anaesthesia. This apparatus has not gained acceptance for routine monitoring, but the cerebral function analysing monitor (CFAM), a later development of the CFM, may be more useful. In addition, this monitor can be used to assess the electrical activity of scalp muscles and evoked potentials can be obtained (Sebel et al., 1983). Unfortunately, the EEG signals seem to relate specifically to each drug given, and each may have a different pattern of activity. The specific problems will not be discussed here, but further progress can be expected in this field.

Stimulation of a peripheral or other nerve can evoke change in the pattern of an EEG, and measurement of this response is the basis of evoked potential analysis, although the analysis is rendered difficult by the presence of normal waves. It is possible by various techniques to eliminate much of this main EEG activity and thus highlight the evoked potentials. They also demonstrate specific linkages of peripheral structures with areas of the brain. The three pathways most extensively studied are the auditory, the somatosensory and the visual. When fully evaluated they offer the promise of a valuable method of assessing depth of anaesthesia.

Other methods of determining the depth of the anaesthetic include oesophageal contractility and the electromyographic (EMG) recordings from the frontalis muscle. The former can be shown as spontaneous waves, which are suppressed during anaesthesia, apparently with a relationship to the depth of the anaesthetic. The latter can detect frowning of a subclinical nature, but they need experience to interpret as the degree of the neuromuscular blockade present also has to be assessed.

### Peripheral nerve stimulators

Incremental doses of the more recently introduced competitive muscle relaxants are frequently given after assessment of the state of the blockade by means of a peripheral nerve stimulator. The more traditional use is to assess the state of the patient immediately before or after reversal at the end of an operation. It is an essential piece of equipment which should also be available in the recovery room.

The exact frequencies and duration of stimuli vary with different instruments and can be varied by the user. A 'train of four' stimulus (four successive stimuli at 2 Hz) is commonly used during anaesthesia to assess the depth of the blockade, although other methods of stimulation, such as 50 Hz tetani, single twitch, double burst stimulation or post-tetanic count all have their advocates for various uses.

### Urine output

During major surgical procedures, when the patient has an indwelling urethral catheter, urinary output provides a guide to renal perfusion, and thus indirectly to the cardiac output. It should be part of the nursing process to note the urine output, both in time and quantity, after any operative or other procedure. In sick patients and after major procedures this should be done accurately, making an indwelling catheter essential. The components of the urine should also be assessed, noting the presence of glucose, ketones or protein. It is important to recognize at an early stage the onset of oliguria, so that treatment can begin and the fluid intake be regulated more closely.

## Historical background

In 1978, the Health Council of the Netherlands sent to the Minister and State Secretary for Health and Environmental Protection an

Advisory Report on Anaesthesiology, later published in 1980. This can probably claim to be the first published paper in the field of monitoring to enhance patient safety (Crul, 1987).

The nine hospitals affiliated to the Harvard Medical School accepted minimum standards of monitoring for all anaesthetized patients (Eichorn *et al.*, 1986) and these were adopted by the American Society of Anesthesiologists House of Delegates in October 1986 (see Table 5.2). In January 1989 similar standards became law in New York State. This meant that every patient who was given a general anaesthetic by means of an endotracheal tube was required to be monitored with an end-tidal carbon dioxide analyser, an inspired oxygen monitor and a disconnection alarm. Later, in February of that year, the State of New Jersey adopted 'Hospital Licensing Standards for Anesthesia Care'. These regulations specify the requirement to have an effective head of department, to adhere to specific standards for certain aspects of machine safety and maintenance schedules, and also for patient monitoring including pulse oximetry and body temperature.

The Faculty of Anaesthetists of the Australian Royal College of Surgeons issued a guide on 'Minimum Facilities for Safe Conduct of Anaesthesia in Operating Suites' in 1984. This was followed by a conference in 1987 where general agreement was reached by Austral-asian anaesthetists on minimal monitoring, as well as critical incident reporting and mortality and morbidity studies. The Australian Patient Safety Foundation was set up (Runciman, 1988).

In the National Health Service in the United Kingdom, the wide disparity in the usage of monitors led to pressure for a more uniform approach. In 1987 an Editorial in the *British Journal of Anaesthesia*, by C. D. Hanning, pleaded for a code of practice for patient monitoring to be instituted. The General Professional Training Guide of the Faculty of Anaesthetists of the Royal College of Surgeons of England was published in 1987, and this document mentioned minimal monitoring. In 1988 the Association of Anaesthetists of Great Britian and Ireland issued their 'Recommendations for the Standard of Monitoring during Anaesthesia and Recovery'. This is an advisory document and is not intended at the present time to compel all anaesthetists to adopt the standards outlined. Table 5.3 shows the main outline of these suggestions. While asserting the fundamental safeguard that the anaesthetist should be present throughout the operation and should not be distracted from clinical observation by other matters, this document is the first attempt in the United Kingdom to apply a standard of monitoring to anaesthesia. Like all such statements this will inevitably lead to these becoming the accepted minimum standards that should be applied to ensure patient care, if not by the profession, then certainly by the courts of law.

In addition to the countries mentioned above, the following have

**Table 5.2    Summary of standards of basic monitoring: American Society of
Anesthesiologists**

---

**Standard 1**    Qualified anesthesia personnel shall be present in the room throughout
the conduct of all general anesthetics, regional anesthetics and monitored
anesthesia care.

**Standard 2.**    During all anesthetics, the patient's oxygenation, ventilation, circulation,
and temperature shall be continually evaluated.

(a) *Oxygenation*
Inspired gas: Oxygen concentration in patient breathing system must be measured
by an analyser with a low limit alarm.
Blood oxygenation: There must be adequate illumination and exposure to assess
patient's colour. Since January 1990 pulse oximetry is mandatory, and more
recently this is also compulsory during immediate post-anesthetic care.

(b) *Ventilation*
Adequacy: Clinical signs, such as chest excursion, observation of the reservoir bag
and auscultation, may be adequate, but monitoring of carbon dioxide content and
expired volume is encouraged.
Placement of endotracheal tube: Must be verified clinically, but the use of end-tidal
carbon dioxide analysis is encouraged. More recently it is obligatory to identify
carbon dioxide in the expired gas.
Mechanical ventilation: A disconnect alarm with an audible signal should be used
continuously.
Regional anesthesia: The adequacy of ventilation should be monitored at least by
continual observation.

(c) *Circulation*
Electrocardiogram: Must be continually displayed from induction until departure
from theatre.
Heart rate and blood pressure: Must be determined and evaluated every 5 minutes.
Monitors: Continual evaluation of the circulation should be provided by at least one
method (palpation of a peripheral pulse, auscultation of the heart sounds, display
of a direct arterial trace, assessment of a peripheral pulse by an ultrasound probe,
pulse plethysmograph or pulse oximetry).

(d) *Temperature*
Measuring device: Should always be available and must be used if a change in body
temperature is anticipated or suspected.

---

also adopted minimum standards of monitoring in the perioperative
period: Canada (1987), Singapore (1988), Belgium (1988), France
(1989), Germany (between 1984 and 1990) and Switzerland (1986
onwards). Worldwide it is thought that at least 12 countries now have
regulations of this type, and although they are not all compulsory by
law, a lack of compliance may invalidate malpractice insurance. In
some countries the regulations extend to the qualifications of the staff
and the facilities provided by the hospital.

In summary, all the recommendations stress the need for continuous
monitoring of the ventilation, oxygenation and circulation, to be
applied not only to all general anaesthetics, but also to regional
anaesthetics, monitored sedation and other anaesthesia care. Although

this process starts with careful clinical observation, it should always be supplemented with the appropriate monitoring devices, some of which are considered to be obligatory in certain countries. Thus, the use of a disconnect alarm when a ventilator is employed, the application of an electrocardiogram (ECG), a noninvasive blood pressure and pulse rate recording at frequent intervals, together with the use of a pulse oximeter and a capnograph, are all becoming a standard requirement for patient monitoring. Other important measurements include the patient's core temperature, the state of neuromuscular block when muscle relaxants are used, and information on the oxygen system.

Debate still centres on the time span and frequency of the measurements. There is general agreement that monitoring should start before induction, and some continuity should be established in the recovery areas until full recovery has occurred, but there is not full agreement about the monitors that are essential postoperatively. The pulse oximeter is probably the most important single monitor, together with clinical observation and recording of pulse rate and blood pressure.

There is some concern that the increased number and type of monitoring devices presently in use, of different shape, design and method of control, with various audible and visible alarms, is not ideal for the operating theatre environment. The displays are not always easily seen by the anaesthetist as they may be placed to one side of the patient or even behind the anaesthetist. This haphazard arrangement of equipment around the anaesthetic machine can lead to mishaps (Winter and Spence, 1990). The mere acquisition of electromedical equipment, perhaps incorrectly applied to the patient for use by staff unfamiliar with it, far from increasing safety, may compound the complexity and confusion around a patient in the operating theatre to such a degree that the reverse ensues.

## Requirements for monitoring worldwide

There are many recommendations for minimum standards of monitoring worldwide, but three groups of recommendations will be compared here. In the United States of America these are those originally propounded by the Harvard Medical School, but afterwards adopted by the American Society of Anesthesiologists. In Australia the recommendations are those of the Faculty of Anaesthetists of the Royal Australasian College of Surgeons which led to the formation of the Australian Patient Safety Foundation. Lastly, in the United Kingdom the recommendations are those published by the Association of Anaesthetists of Great Britain and Ireland (Winter and Spence, 1990). There seems to be little difference in these three sets of propositions, and the recommendations fall into five groups. (See also Tables 5.2 and 5.3.)

Table 5.3    Summary of standards of monitoring: Association of Anaesthetists of Great Britain and Ireland

| | |
|---|---|
| (a) | Anaesthetist should be continuously present and make an adequate record. |
| (b) | Monitoring should start before induction and continue until recovery is complete. |
| (c) | The anaesthetic machine should be monitored by an oxygen analyser with alarms and a disconnection alarm. |
| (d) | Continuous monitoring of ventilation and circulation is essential. This should be by clinical observation supplemented by monitoring devices. |
| (e) | Frequency of blood pressure and pulse rate measurements should be appropriate to the state of the patient. |
| (f) | A peripheral nerve stimulator should be available when muscle relaxants are employed. |
| (g) | Long or complicated operations and sick patients may require additional monitoring. |
| (h) | Adequate monitoring is required during brief operations, and during procedures under local anaesthetic and sedation. |
| (i) | Appropriate monitoring should be used during the transport of a patient. |
| (j) | Adequate instructions concerning monitoring should be given to recovery ward staff, and appropriate monitors should be available. |

## Minimal monitoring standards

### 1   The anaesthetist

There is a requirement for the continuous presence of a properly qualified anaesthetist. An essential part of his or her duties is to ensure adequate ventilation by observation of the motion of the reservoir bag and the patient's chest wall. The anaesthetist should also continuously assess the cardiac output by observing the patient's colour and capillary refill time and noting the character and rate of the pulse.

### 2   Simple monitoring

The patient should be connected to an ECG and a noninvasive method of blood pressure measurement, and this presumably means from before induction until full recovery. The ECG is not considered essential in Australia. In the United States and Australia it is now essential to apply a pulse oximeter, and many anaesthetists in the United Kingdom would also employ this instrument in every case.

### 3   Machine monitors

It is considered essential that the anaesthetic machine should have a ventilator disconnection alarm and a means of analysing the inspired oxygen. A low inspired oxygen alarm is obligatory in the United States. In Australia and the United Kingdom it is also considered essential to have a warning for failure of the oxygen supply.

### 4   Patient monitors

It is recommended, but not essential, to have a pulse oximeter in the United Kingdom, but it is mandatory in the other two countries. An end-tidal carbon dioxide analyser is also recommended in intubated patients, and in the United States a means of identifying expired carbon dioxide is considered essential – of the available methods, the capnograph is the ideal. All three countries recognize the value of spirometry, but it is classified as recommended equipment only in the United States and the United Kingdom. Other means of monitoring specific parameters should be available at the discretion of the anaesthetist.

### 5   Essential supplementary equipment

Three pieces of equipment should be available in the operating theatre complex if the anaesthetist requires them. These are: appropriate temperature probes, a peripheral nerve stimulator and a means of direct invasive pressure monitoring, both for arterial and venous use. Invasive blood pressure monitoring is almost mandatory for a major procedure. The peripheral nerve stimulator is not considered important in the United States. Clearly the anaesthetist is responsible for applying the discretionary apparatus in the appropriate patients.

In both the United Kingdom and Australia a brief operation on a patient whose physical status is ASA grade I requires continuous clinical monitoring of ventilation and circulation, which should be supplemented by at least an ECG and a noninvasive blood pressure apparatus. The use of the pulse oximeter and capnograph is strongly recommended (Winter and Spence, 1990). In addition, the anaesthetic machine used should have an oxygen supply failure warning device, and if IPPV is contemplated it should also have a ventilator disconnection alarm. The Harvard Medical School system, which is the basis for the American Society of Anesthesiologists' recommendations, is in some States embodied in Statute Law (Eichorn et al., 1986). There is still debate as to whether these measures have affected patient outcome (see Chapter 8), but there is no doubt that the various bodies that provide indemnity are satisfied they do indeed increase patient safety.

## Recording the observations

It has been traditional for anaesthetists to fill in a 'chart' during the course of an operation. This activity is often undertaken in a casual and untidy way, and has never been thought of as compulsory. It is also quite clear that these records must have been compiled after events they describe, and indeed are often subjected to revision when rewriting a chart for perfectly legitimate reasons. During critical times the delay in recording may be greater, and the information is not infrequently incomplete or inaccurate. These charts are intended as an *aide-mémoire* to those charged with the postoperative care, and also for future anaesthetics. A subsidiary use may be in research.

It is, however, unfortunate that if the patient to whom these documents relate becomes party to a legal enquiry or court case, the records are closely scrutinized by the lawyers concerned; they are then treated far more seriously than perhaps their origins warrant. It would seem that more care is required in the writing of these documents, especially in the statements made, the timings given and the doses stated. The charting of the results of the functions measured is frequently deplorable. A much wider use should be made of recorders with a real time capability to record the blood pressure, heart rate, temperature and possibly respiratory rate on hard copy. In addition, other measurements should be added manually if the machine is not capable of printing them. These include oxygen saturation, end-tidal carbon dioxide, inspired oxygen and volatile agents.

It is not within the scope of this book to set standards of charting, but it is clear that the present methods do not produce a useful document in many cases. When handwritten records are compared with monitor records in the same patient, many discrepancies are found (Cook, McDonald and Nunziata, 1989). It is likely that in the near future automated records will be produced and may even be regarded in the same way as the 'black box' information in aviation, although the record of the anaesthetic will not be erased at the end of the procedure as in the commercial field (Lees, 1990). The ultimate development could be a 'medical information bus', where the anaesthetic information will form but one part of a totally integrated, computer controlled system.

If an untoward event occurs this merits a full note of all the circumstances together with a proper chart of the patient's functions. It is quite permissible to do this after first taking the urgent actions required for the health and safety of the patient, but a note of the time of writing is essential, together with an indication of the measurements which are certain and if possible capable of verification. Since the document may become the subject of legal scrutiny, a list of those people present and their status is important and should be added.

# References

American Society of Anesthesiologists House of Delegates (1986) *Standards for Basic Intra-operative Monitoring*, Park Ridge, Ill., ASA, 21 October 1986

Andersen, K. H. and Hald, A. (1989) Assessing the position of the tracheal tube. The reliability of different methods. *Anaesthesia*, **44**, 984–985

Association of Anaesthetists of Great Britain and Ireland (1988) *Recommendations for the Standard of Monitoring During Anaesthesia and Recovery*, London

Brahams, D. (1989) Anaesthesia and the law: monitoring. *Anaesthesia*, **44**, 606–607

Brice, D. D., Hetherington, R. R. and Utting, J. E. (1970) A simple study of awareness and dreaming during anaesthesia. *British Journal of Anaesthesia*, **42**, 535–541

Cook, R. I., McDonald, J. S. and Nunziata, E. (1989) Differences between handwritten and automatic blood pressure records. *Anesthesiology*, **71**, 385–390

Crul, J. F. (1987) The Netherlands national approach to standards of safety and care in anesthesia. *European Journal of Anaesthesiology*, **4**, 213–215

Eichorn, J. H., Cooper, J. B., Cullen, D. J., Maier, W. R., Philip, J. H. and Seeman, R. G. (1986) Standards for patient monitoring at Harvard Medical School. *JAMA*, **256**, 1017–1020

Faculty of Anaesthetists, Royal Australasian College of Surgeons (1984) *Minimum Facilities for Safe Conduct of Anaesthesia in Operating Suites*, RACS

Faculty of Anaesthetists, Royal College of Surgeons of England (1987) *General Professional Training Guide*, RCS, London

Foëx, P. and Prys-Roberts, C. (1974) Anaesthesia and the hypertensive patient. *British Journal of Anaesthesia*, **46**, 575–588

Hanning, C. D. (1987) Editorial: Monitoring – bane or blessing? *British Journal of Anaesthesia*, **59**, 1201–1202

Hargrove, R. L. (1987) Awareness under anaesthesia. *Journal of the Medical Defence Union*, **3**, 9–11

Health Technical Memorandum (1972) *Piped Medical Gases, Compressed Air and Medical Vacuum Installations*, Department of Health, London, 22 May, 1972, revised June 1990

Ilsley, A. H., Plummer, J. L., Runciman, W. B. and Cousins, M. J. (1986) An evaluation of three volatile anaesthetic monitors. *Anaesthesia and Intensive Care*, **14**, 431–436

Lees, D. E. (1990) Anesthesiology equipment – the next decade, the next century. *American Society of Anesthesiologists Newsletter*, **54**, 4–7

Memorandum (1977) Oxygen supply pressure failure warning and protection devices. *Anaesthesia*, **31**, 316

Pryn, S. J. and Cross, M. M. (1989) Ventilator disconnection alarm failure. *Anaesthesia*, **44**, 978–981

Runciman, W. B. (1988) The Australian Patient Safety Foundation. *Anaesthesia and Intensive case*, **16**, 114–116

Runciman, W. B., Rutten, A. J. and Ilsley, A. H. (1981) An evaluation of blood pressure measurement. *Anaesthesia and Intensive Care*, **9**, 314–325

Sebel, P. S., Maynard, D. E., Major, E. and Frank, M. (1983) The cerebral function analysing monitor (CFAM): a new microprocessor based device for an on-line EEG and evoked potential analysis. *British Journal of Anaesthesia*, **55**, 1265–1270

Swan, H. J. C., Ganz, W., Forrester, J. S., Marcus, H., Diamond, G. and Chonette, D. (1970) Catheterization of the heart in man with the use of a flow-directed balloon-tipped catheter. *New England Journal of Medicine*, **283**, 447–451

Sykes, M. K. (1987) Essential monitoring. *British Journal of Anaesthesia*, **59**, 901–912

Taylor, M. B. and Whitwam, J. G. (1986) The current status of pulse oximetry. *Anaesthesia*, **41**, 943–949

Wee, M. Y. K. (1988) The oesophageal detector device. *Anaesthesia*, **43**, 27–29

Weingarten, M. (1986) Anesthetic and ventilator mishaps: prevention and detection. *Critical Care Medicine*, **14**, 1084

Winter, A. and Spence, A. A. (1990) Editorial: An international consensus on monitoring? *British Journal of Anaesthesia*, **64**, 263–266

# 6

# Care of staff and the working environment

This book describes what the authors believe to be appropriate standards of care for a patient undergoing anaesthesia. The present chapter, while still recognizing this remit, now proceeds to review the equipment and standards of care which ensure that the activities of the anaesthetist, and to a lesser extent of the surgeon, do not endanger the welfare of the theatre and hospital staff, some of whom may not be directly involved with the patient in question. Measures to improve the welfare of the staff, such as the use of scavenging apparatus to remove waste anaesthetic gases, could conflict with the best interest of the patient if not properly installed and carefully used. Thus some procedures and apparatus introduced to protect the health and safety of the hospital staff may present an unforeseen hazard for the patient. It is the duty of those that introduce these arrangements to ensure that the welfare of the patient remains paramount.

There are seven areas for concern when attempting to prevent harm to the patient and hospital staff from environmental hazards in the operating theatre, and these are shown in Table 6.1. Three are related

**Table 6.1  Protection of patients and staff from environmental hazards**

Equipment-related factors
1. Removal of anaesthetic gases from the atmosphere
2. Disposal of used syringes, needles and 'sharps'
3. Control of infection
    (a) Patient
    (b) Staff

Staff-related factors
1. Environmental temperature and humidity
2. Fatigue and stress
3. Noise
4. Drug and alcohol abuse

to the apparatus and materials used by the anaesthetist and surgeon, and four are controls and regulations necessary to maintain the efficiency of the staff working in the operating theatre. The latter do have a direct influence on patient care, however, because they all relate to the working conditions and environent of the staff, and the staff have to be at peak efficiency at all times in the stressful circumstances of the operating theatre and recovery areas if the care given to the patient is to be optimal.

# Equipment-related factors

## Removal of waste anaesthetic gases from the atmosphere

This process is popularly known as 'scavenging', and is now the subject of regulation by government agencies and comes within the Control of Substances Hazardous to Health regulations. The basis for this requirement is the impression that staff working in an atmosphere containing halogenated anaesthetic vapour and nitrous oxide are subject to health hazards, and much effort has been expanded in attempts to define a causal relationship, especially with regard to the outcome of pregnancy. These attempts have not clearly demonstrated such a relationship, and final conclusions must await the results of large prospective enquiries, such as that of Knill-Jones and Spence, who started collection of ten-year data in 1977, thus finishing in 1986. Their early conclusions show no obvious association between environmental waste gases and the outcome of pregnancy in women in these areas (Spence, Wall and Nunn, 1989).

Early workers sought information from respondents on the incidence of spontaneous abortion and congenital anomalies. The responses seemed to suggest that females and the wives of males working in these areas suffered a higher than normal rate of infertility and spontaneous abortion. It was also thought that this group of hospital workers might have a higher incidence of congenital malformations in their offspring. None of these allegations has been conclusively proved in prospective controlled investigations, although Vessey and Nunn (1980) comprehensively reviewed the literature and concluded that there was an increased risk of spontaneous abortion. It is difficult to be sure that this is not simply reporting bias, and there was no firm evidence of other reported sequelae. Other work suggested that the evidence for a health hazard is unreliable (Pharoah et al., 1977; Tannenbaum and Goldberg, 1985). Buring et al., in 1985, examining 17 published studies on the subject of theatre pollution and combining the data from six that were thought to be statistically reliable, concluded that the most consistent adverse outcome was spontaneous abortion in pregnant females working in the operating room. The relative risk was 30% greater than the control population. They did, however, point out the limitation of their conclusions, in that nine of the 17 papers considered were eliminated because of deficiencies in the design of the studies. Even the six studies examined had some deficiencies, notably the absence of medical verification of the medical outcomes reported in the questionnaires, and the degree of 'exposure' in the group alleged to have been subject to the health hazard (Mazze, 1985).

It was also suspected that those who worked in a polluted environment had a higher rate of lymphatic and other tumours. This also has not been confirmed subsequently, although animal studies still lend some support to the idea. In both the United Kingdom and the United States there is an increased incidence of hepatitis in anaesthetists (Cohen et al., 1974; Buring et al., 1985). Halothane can depress the liver function on chronic exposure to low concentrations, and a few isolated cases of hepatitis have been reported in anaesthetists (Stock and Strunin, 1985). Exclusion from an atmosphere polluted with halothane leads to a reversal of the condition.

Of all the pollutants known to exist in the theatre atmosphere, the adverse metabolic effects of nitrous oxide is best documented. It oxidizes the cobalt ion in vitamin $B_{12}$, and therefore interferes with DNA synthesis. Long-term exposure may thus result in several disabilities, including megaloblastic anaemia, leucopenia, peripheral neuropathy and possibly fetal damage. Extrapolating from exposure studies on rats, it is thought that a safe exposure level in the operating theatre environment lies below 450 parts per million. There is no effect on methionine synthesis within this range. This is a high pollution level, even in an unscavenged theatre, and it is unlikely that staff would be exposed to this concentration continuously throughout the working day. Such a level could be found in dental surgeries continually using the gas as an analgesic in conservation work, which takes a considerable time to perform, and cases of abnormalities have been reported in the practitioners of this type of dentistry (Sweeney et al., 1985). Nitrous oxide causes megaloblastic changes and leucopenia after prolonged exposure and also after short-term exposure (Nunn, Sharer and Gorschein, 1982). Again there is no consistent evidence of a harmful effect on theatre personnel in the normal course of their work, where routine operating lists are undertaken (Spence, 1987). Peripheral neuropathy has been reported in persons who have inhaled nitrous oxide for long periods, probably as a form of drug abuse (Layzer, Fishman and Schafter, 1978).

The trauma of surgery is a significant factor in observed postoperative immunosuppression of previously normal individuals, and is probably more important than the anaesthetic agents concurrently employed. There is no doubt, however, that anaesthetic agents also suppress the response and this may be important in patients already compromised, such as those suffering from AIDS or cancer. Despite this effect when anaesthetic concentrations of vapours are employed, theatre and anaesthetic personnel do not appear to be at risk from traces found in the atmosphere in their working environment (Salo and Vapaavuori, 1976).

From the patient's point of view, however, the most important effect of atmospheric pollution was shown by Bruce and his co-workers in 1974. This followed previous work by the same author in conjunction with Linde (1969). The latter work found that anaesthetists had recognizable amounts of halothane and nitrous oxide in their end-expired gases. The wash-out time for these is as long as 64 hours, which means that the pollutant gases are cumulative for individuals in the context of the hours currently worked by most theatre staff and anaesthetists, for a 2 day/3 night weekend is needed for the complete clearance of these gases. The 1974 paper showed that traces of anaesthetic gases in workers in operating theatres affected their performance, especially in skilled manipulations. This is similar to the effect of alcohol, and is therefore not unexpected. But if the level of atmospheric pollution was persistently high, the rate of error could become unacceptable. It should not be necessary to remind the reader that many studies have shown that the majority of avoidable anaesthetic mishaps are caused by human error. It therefore follows that any conditions that may increase the chance of such a mishap must be avoided, and this is the justification for the extra risk to the patient that the use of scavenging apparatus may impose.

Thus, although the emphasis in the literature is on waste anaesthetic gases, there is no conclusive evidence that they cause harm to the theatre staff. Moreover, these persons are also subjected to many other vapours, some of which may be harmful. They include methylmethacrylate and various alcohols and other solvents. They are also subject to radiation hazards, infective particles and, perhaps more importantly, to stress, which can on occasions be severe.

At the present time the evidence that the scavenging of waste anaesthetic gases significantly benefits the theatre staff is equivocal. Therefore it would seem that the use of scavenging apparatus can only be justified if there is virtually no added risk to the safety of the patient. Overall safety may be enhanced if available money is channelled into other safety measures. Nevertheless it should be noted that various bodies world wide have issued scavenging standards.

The Association of Anaesthetists of Great Britain and Ireland first suggested the use of scavenging equipment in this country in 1975. Although the dangers were brought to the attention of the health authorities, no strict guidance was issued. In 1987 a British Standard was given for the performance of scavenging systems (BS 6834:1987).

In the United States precise levels of gases permitted in the operating theatre environment were laid down (NIOSH, 1977). The concentration of nitrous oxide should not exceed 25 parts per million, and for the halogenated vapours 2 parts per million or 0.5 parts per million when used together with nitrous oxide. These levels could probably only be achieved with fastidious attention to detail and very efficient scavenging devices, and it is probable that they represent too high a standard.

The apparatus used to reduce the levels to those desired will not be described here. A useful account can be found in 'Anaesthetic Equipment' by C. S. Ward (1985). In principle, the gases are ducted to the outside air, either passively through a low resistance piping system or actively by a negative pressure on the patient circuit. The use of this apparatus introduces hazards to the patient, and anaesthetists must be familiar with these and protect their patients from the unwanted effects. The use of flammable anaesthetics has declined dramatically in the developed countries, but they should not be used with most scavenging systems, since most incorporate non-antistatic materials, may be driven electrically and the eventual waste outlet may be unprotected from casual ignition, for example by a discarded cigarette end. It is also important to ensure that the hose carrying the effluent away from the patient's scavenging valve is never obstructed.

Protection from pressure build-up is afforded in scavenging circuits by incorporating a 'break' in the system, but it is not possible to place these in close proximity to the patient and some connecting hose is required before the break. The distal part of the system is then rendered safe, for any obstruction in this part will not lead to an excessive rise of pressure in the patient's lungs, but the connecting hose near the patient remains vulnerable.

It should be realized that the use of scavenging apparatus is not the only method for reducing the levels of pollutants in the atmosphere. The quantity of gas escaping into the theatre environment can be limited by other means. Although theatre air-conditioning systems are not designed to remove pollutants, but to maintain an equable temperature and humidity while minimizing bacterial contamination, an adequate ventilation system will change the air frequently. The actual volume of waste gases released can be reduced by using low flow circuits and putting a greater emphasis on regional and intravenous techniques. All apparatus should be regularly tested for leaks, and the flowmeters and vaporizers must be turned off at the end of a case. Vaporizers should be filled with care to avoid spillage of the liquid agent, and this should be done outside the operating theatre.

Postoperatively, when patients are in the recovery room or an intensive care unit after receiving an anaesthetic containing nitrous oxide and halogenated agents, the gases are expired into the atmosphere in measurable quantities for several hours. There is at present no satisfactory apparatus that can be used in these areas unless the patient is intubated. Most available apparatus is in the form of a 'tent', and is not only dangerous because it prohibits close nursing attention, but is terrifying to the patient when he becomes aware of his surroundings. Recovery rooms and intensive care units should have ventilation systems capable of at least twenty air changes each hour. If the atmosphere is polluted above an acceptable level, the staff may have to be re-rostered to shorten the hours of exposure of each individual.

The protection of the environment in areas where inhalational anaesthesia is given in the dental chair is also difficult, for there are design problems with apparatus because of the lack of an airtight system to deliver the anaesthetic in those patients who are not intubated. Greater emphasis on intravenous techniques would help to reduce the overall levels, but again reliance has to be placed on frequent air changes in the room by the ventilating system and ensuring the staff are not continuously exposed for prolonged periods. Leakage directly from the apparatus and spillage of the liquid agents are again an important source of pollution.

Although the general assumption is that the atmosphere in all parts of the operating theatre has a consistent general level of pollutant gases, this clearly is not so, as the vapours will disperse at a lower concentration throughout the room from the high level leakage source. Personnel near an unscavenged expiratory valve are likely to inhale a higher concentration and thus to attain higher blood levels than those further away. This variation in different parts of the operating theatre makes it virtually impossible to sample the atmosphere in any satisfactory way from one point, unless a 'sampler' is attached directly to the member of staff most at risk. If monitoring is thought to be essential, it is probably best achieved from end-tidal samples of personnel or by taking blood samples for analysis from individual staff members most at risk.

## The disposal of used syringes, needles and sharps

The term 'sharps' is a colloquial expression, which now seems to be accepted in normal usage, to cover a range of detritus, from used scalpel blades and stilettes to glass from ampoules. It is reasonable to discuss these various pieces together as they all have the capability of inflicting puncture wounds to the staff that handle them. The possibility of this happening of course extends to those nonskilled staff engaged on the disposal of hospital refuse. To ensure the full protection of these workers, whose knowledge of the dangers of the materials they are handling may be minimal, must be a prime concern of the users and the hospital management.

Many of these discarded items have been in contact with body fluids, especially blood, which may be infected. The possibility of transferring infection varies with the nature of the organism present.

The chance of transferring HIV has been shown to be remote, but four cases have been reported showing accidental inoculation of blood from a previously used hollow needle. (Editorial, 1984). A further 15 cases have been reported by Roger *et al.* in 1989. The possibility of infection of health care workers is greater with the virus of hepatitis B, and this occurs with inoculation incidents or contamination of skin (Tedder, 1983). It is therefore important to protect all staff from the possibility of a puncture wound, and this includes those outside the theatre complex who man the waste disposal services. Clearly protective gloves should be worn by these people, but anaesthetists and their assistants should place potentially dangerous articles in a stout container, the walls of which are incapable of being pierced by the contents, and these containers with their contents should be incinerated before ultimate disposal. The hospital should collect such potentially dangerous waste separately from the normal domestic rubbish, use special measures for its removal until it can be made safe by incineration and ensure that it is eventually deposited in a proper place.

The British Medical Association's Board of Science has produced a 'Code of Practice on the Safe Use and Disposal of Sharps' (British Medical Association, 1990) in response to the increasing incidence of injuries from these objects. Although there are at least 22 blood-borne pathogens that may cause infection, the main danger comes from HIV and the hepatitis B virus. The code recommends that sharps should be placed in a safe bin immediately after use and the needle should never be resheathed. The syringe and needle should be discarded together, and not left lying around. It also contains information on risk management and procedures to be adopted if an injury occurs.

'Needle-stick' injuries are most feared by staff, as it is perceived that this is a possible route of infection with HIV, although the virus of hepatitis B is more dangerous. It is thought that the former cannot be acquired through the intact skin and a considerable inoculum is required to initiate infection, making a needle essential. This is probably not true of the latter. If substantial (greater than 1 ml) amounts of blood are thought to be injected after a needle-stick injury, or if the puncture was definitely parenteral (intramuscular or deep), it is recommended that prophylactic zidovudine should be started without delay, if possible within 2 hours of injury. The drug is known to have considerable side effects. Safety could be enhanced if apparatus were designed to be used without the need for a needle when giving a drug to a patient, for example by the use of ports in the intravenous line to which the syringe can be directly attached. In this way only one sharp needle would be contaminated for each case, that used for the initial entry into the patient's bloodstream.

The glass ampoules containing drugs are a source of danger, especially if they fracture, and should be opened with care. Plastic containers are now available. If in general use, they could obviate this hazard.

## The control of infection

### The patient

Within the confines of this present book it is impossible to survey the measures required to ensure that infections are controlled in the operating theatre from the surgical point of view. Our account will be limited to the measures needed to ensure that the apparatus used by the anaesthetist is made safe.

When anaesthesia is induced and the patient prepared for surgery, the anaesthetist is engaged in work in a potentially infected area – the mouth and upper airway – while he or she is also gaining access to the vascular system for intravenous therapy and monitoring. It should be clear that these two main areas of activity must be separated in time and the materials used from different work-tops in order to prevent contamination. If a regional or local anaesthetic is to be employed in addition, even more care should be exercised. The operator should wash his hands between procedures as well as between patients. Gloves should preferably be worn for most procedures and work surfaces should be cleaned with a bacteriocidal solution between each activity.

Despite possible contamination with the patient's own organisms from the mouth and upper airway, all apparatus that comes into contact with the patient's airway below the vocal cords should be sterile at the beginning of an anaesthetic, for it is easy to introduce infection into the lungs by this means. This is especially important in sick patients and those who are immunologically compromised. The sterilization of rubber apparatus is difficult, and in many services this has been replaced by pre-packed disposable plastic equipment, usually sterilized by gamma-radiation. The dose of gamma-radiation required to destroy bacteria is 2.5 megarads, usually from a cobalt 60 device. The dose is applied through the external packing. The availability of single-use endotracheal tubes and catheter mounts, often including a humidification device, is almost universal, and disposable circuits are becoming more common in the United Kingdom. Their use obviates the need for considerable work in the theatre sterile supplies unit, and also the expensive special apparatus to clean them. Unless the patient is of special risk, cleaning and washing the circuits frequently, without absolute sterility, is sufficient to prevent an infection being transmitted from one patient to another (Nielsen, Vasegaard and Stokes, 1978).

The anaesthetic face mask is the most difficult part of the delivery apparatus to clean. This is because the rubber air cushion cannot be heat-sterilized. In any case heat markedly shortens the useful life of antistatic rubber. This means that masks have to be carefully washed in soapy water and dried. The use of chemical detergents must be avoided because they cause skin sensitivity and may get into the eyes. Disposable masks are available and are used extensively in the United States, but are not used widely in the United Kingdom. It would seem likely that in the future they will be used more.

Metal articles can be heat or chemically sterilized, provided the latter agents are removed subsequently by repeated rinsing. The advent of fibreoptic light systems has made this process possible with laryngoscopes, because the detachable blade has no electric bulb in it, and can be soaked in sterilizing solution or heat-treated to a limited temperature.

In the developed countries the apparatus required for vascular access and monitoring, as well as that used for local anaesthetic techniques, is now universally of the 'single-use' kind, sterilized by gamma-radiation and pre-packed. In circumstances where the use of this type of material is not possible, the individual practitioner must take responsibility for ensuring that the methods used by his assistants are satisfactory and result in sterile equipment which causes no damage to the patient. Local anaesthetic and other drugs used for regional techniques are especially important, and in the developed countries these are now supplied in individual sterile packs, which have again been sterilized by gamma-radiation.

Anaesthetic and intensive care ventilators present a special problem when they need to be sterilized. Many now incorporate a patient's circuit which is detachable and autoclavable, or use disposable patient circuits. This still leaves some areas of the machine which are inaccessible to normal methods, and many ways of sterilizing them have been described. Ventilators, as well as the conventional anaesthetic machine, can be protected to some extent from bacterial contamination by the use of suitable filters. This is especially valuable with ventilators which entrain room air into the patient's circuit. It is necessary to change them at prescribed intervals, for a heavily contaminated filter becomes a dangerous source of infection.

### The staff

There are some infections encountered in hospital practice which require more specific precautions when the sufferer presents for operation, mainly for the protection of the staff but also to protect any patient who is operated upon subsequently in the same theatre. The infective agents include HIV, hepatitis B, herpes simplex, tubercle, *Pseudomonas pyocyanea*, all infections with antibiotic-resistant organisms and Creutzfeldt–Jakob disease. Further information can be obtained from *Control of Hospital Infection* by Lowbury *et al.* (1981).

Individual institutions will have their own policies to be applied when patients suffering from these infections undergo surgery. Most of these include removal of all apparatus not immediately required from the infected area. This means that the anaesthetist must make sure that all essential equipment is available before the patient is induced, and that he has an assistant available immediately outside the theatre with a knowledge of the storage position of any item that might be required urgently.

All the staff involved with these cases should wear disposable gloves, masks and suits. The provision of eye shields is essential for those at most risk, for example from a patient coughing, and becomes even more important when power tools are being employed, for these cause a fine droplet spray of potentially infected particles in the immediate vicinity of the operation.

In a study by Harrison and co-workers (1990), it was shown that blood had contaminated the skin of a total of 65 anaesthetic staff on 46 occasions. This blood came from 35 patients, 14% of the total studied. Sixty-one per cent of the incidents arose during cannulation of a vessel, and 8% of the staff had cuts on their hands at this time. There were far fewer incidents of contamination with saliva. Of those involved in the study, 71% were immunized against hepatitis B. Hepatitis B can also be transmitted through the conjunctiva, and there are theoretical reasons for believing that HIV can be transmitted in a similar way. The risk of blood contaminating the eye of the surgeon or anaesthetist is especially likely in arterial and gastrointestinal surgery, and in operations of a long duration, and therefore eye protection may be necessary in this type of work. All theatre staff should receive immunity, certainly on a voluntary basis. The study also showed that gloves were not worn universally, and the importance of this form of protection cannot be over-emphasized.

The Royal College of Surgeons of England stated recently that although HIV is not easily transmitted during surgical procedures, and it is improbable that it can penetrate intact skin, there is a risk present (Royal College of Surgeons, 1990). Infection with HIV from a 'sharps' injury is less than 0.5%, whereas the risk of acquiring hepatitis B with a similar injury is 20%. Needle-stick injuries are the predominant cause throughout the world. In contrast there has been no record of transmission of HIV from a health worker to a patient in the United Kingdom. The College concludes by suggesting that routine testing of all patients is unnecessary at the present time, although desirable in certain high risk groups. They nevertheless feel that a surgeon who is injured during the treatment of a high risk case should have the right to test the patient's status without his consent, and the patient informed after the operation. This advice is contrary to that given by the British Medical Association, but seems to the present authors to be realistic.

# Staff-related factors

## Environmental temperature and humidity

In addition to the patient, whose welfare is paramount at all times, there are three groups of individuals also present in the operating theatre who require a comfortable environment to perform their work well. These three groups are the surgeons and the scrub nurse, the anaesthetist and his assistant and the general theatre staff. The environmental temperature and to a lesser extent the humidity required by each group differs, and therefore the final theatre environment must be a compromise for all three, provided the result is suitable for the patient.

First it is essential to prevent both heat and water vapour loss by the patient. Heat loss is a particular problem in theatres in which laminar flow is fitted, which are mainly used for joint replacement surgery. The prevention of heat and water vapour loss would normally require a high theatre ambient temperature and humidity. Since this would be above that acceptable to the staff, local means of warming the patient are employed, such as warm water blankets. Inspired gases from the cylinders or pipeline are absolutely dry, and water vapour, and therefore heat, are lost with the expired gas. This loss can be reduced considerably by using low gas flows in a circuit with carbon dioxide absorption. If full gas flows are used a heat and moisture exchanger connected to the patient circuit close to the endotracheal tube will minimize the loss of water vapour but not of heat, as this will be necessary to vaporize the condensed water again on re-entry into the lungs. Thus water loss from the patient's lungs is reduced, and perhaps the heat loss is slightly reduced. Against these modest advantages must be set the increased risk of disconnection, the significant increase in resistance to flow in the exchanger if it becomes wet, and the cost of the disposable apparatus. Similarly loss of heat from open body cavities can be minimized by protecting the surfaces with warm saline packs. The fluids that are transfused should also be warmed to body temperature. In prolonged operations or in children, where heat loss can be great and rapid, use can be made of lightweight foil blankets to wrap the parts of the body away from the operative field. The heat loss through an unprotected head can be large, especially in neonates. The ambient temperature of the operating theatre should be raised for children, despite the needs of the surgeon and scrub nurse.

As long ago as 1968, Wyon, Lidwell and Williams showed that anaesthetists preferred a warmer environment to surgeons. The surgeons wear an extra layer of clothes and are in close proximity to the theatre light which gives out considerable heat. It is important that the surgeons should not have to work in an atmosphere so warm as to cause them to perspire profusely, for this could be a factor in the spread of infection. A simple solution would be the use of an extra layer of clothes by the anaesthetist and others in the general theatre team. The problem is acute in theatres which have high air-flow systems moving away from the operating table to preserve the sterile air field around the operating site, as are commonly employed for orthopaedic procedures such as joint replacement. This system gives rise to the movement of large volumes of air, which although warmed to a reasonable temperature, feel very cold to those exposed to the flow.

The most recent regulations from the Department of Health and Social Security (1983) include precautions regarding loss of heat from the patient because of high air-flow devices and the control of noise pollution from these systems. Noise pollution is also referred to below.

## Fatigue and stress

Modern surgery and anaesthesia requires strict attention to detail and close application to many intricate processes. The provision of apparatus to monitor various parameters clearly aids the anaesthetist in this task. Continuous detailed work of this kind must lead to fatigue. (Green, 1986). Comparison has been drawn between the similarity of these activities and those of an airline pilot, not only in this aspect, but also with regard to the need for continuous 'cockpit drill'. The work of the pilot is very closely controlled, both in procedural matters and in respect of hours worked, shift patterns and rostering. It has been suggested that there could be applications for similar forms of organization among people working in a theatre environment. Similarly, it has been suggested that the use of simulators could provide better training for anaesthetists for the critical incidents that occur somewhat rarely in the course of an otherwise uneventful anaesthetic.

There is evidence that many hospital staff, especially the doctors in training, do indeed work long hours. Common sense would infer that this could lead to some failure of attention and subsequently to problems for the patient (Wallace-Barnhill et al., 1983). Anaesthetic departments have been in the forefront in recognizing this when producing on-call rotas. Unfortunately, although the paramount role of human error in producing anaesthetic mishaps is acknowledged, fatigue has not been shown consistently to be the cause. Human error seems to be due either to lack of knowledge through inexperience, or to lack of clinical observation. The work of Bruce, Back and Arbit (1974) elucidating the effects of traces of waste anaesthetic gases in the theatre atmosphere has already been mentioned, but should again be noted in this context.

It has been shown that interrupted sleep patterns impair the response of doctors to procedures which they would normally find easy (Hawkins et al., 1985). Anaesthetists frequently find themselves subjected to sleep deprivation, as much emergency surgery is performed out of normal working hours. The necessity for this night work should be closely scrutinized in all hospitals with a view to postponing non-urgent events to the next day. Where a significant night work load is essential the rosters should allow the duty anaesthetist adequate time off on the following day to recover. The cumulative effect of the deprivation of sleep and irregular food intake has been implicated in causing depression and other stress-related conditions, especially as the specialty is of itself of a kind that can cause periods of acute anxiety about a particular anaesthetic problem. This has been examined in detail in house officers by Firth-Cozens (1989).

The Department of Health (1990) has agreed to ensure that doctors in training are not compelled to undertake excessive continuous on-call commitments. Their maximum duty is to be limited to 72 hours per week, and adequate rest is to be ensured after a period on continuous duty at night.

## Noise

When individuals are closely engaged in work that is technically difficult, or requires close concentration on small details, intrusive noise can add to the stress and fatigue suffered by the individual. Safety dictates that it is essential to maintain some audible alarms, for both anaesthetic monitors and surgical apparatus such as diathermy machines. The initial alarm sounds should be relatively quiet and not of an unpleasant nature. Further alarm events must, of course, produce a noise level that ensures a response from the theatre staff nearby, and thus inevitably be more intrusive and louder if they are to fulfil their function.

Other sounds commonly heard in the operating theatre are not essential and should be silenced. Included in these are irrelevant conversations, telephone bells or buzzers and hospital paging systems. It should be possible for the last two to be intercepted outside the operating theatre, and messages relayed at a time which is convenient so as not to distract the attention of the surgeon and anaesthetist from the essential task of caring for the patient. It is quite unacceptable for loud alarm bells, warning of fire or cardiovascular collapse elsewhere, to intrude into the quiet calm of a well-regulated operating theatre. Other arrangements should be made to intercept these essential warnings and relay them in an appropriate manner.

'Machinery' noise is also distracting. This can come from suction apparatus, gas and scavenging systems, as well as the activities of staff preparing instruments. All these sounds should be kept to a minimum, by installing high quality machinery initially, and by enforcing proper maintenance.

## Drug and alcohol abuse

Anaesthetists are statistically very prone to abuse drugs and alcohol. While the problem is not uncommon in the medical profession at large, the easy access that anaesthetists have to controlled drugs and the anaesthetic gases and vapours make it inevitable that a greater number are at risk.

The practice of anaesthesia can on occasions be very stressful, especially when a tragic mishap occurs, and this is another factor in increasing the risk of drug abuse. The solitary nature of the work may lead to delay in the diagnosis, and thus place patients at great risk, for they are all too often dependent for their wellbeing on the ability and acumen of the individual so affected. It must therefore be the duty of all hospital staff to be alert to the problem of drug and alcohol abuse in their colleagues. If suspicion is aroused action should be taken quickly, for the consequences to the patient of an anaesthetist incapable through drink or drugs are terrifying. Obviously early access to treatment is also desirable for the affected anaesthetist.

The problem was highlighted when the addiction of a consultant anaesthetist to anaesthetic vapours led to the death of a child, because the airway was not properly maintained. In the United Kingdom, the Association of Anaesthetists introduced an Early Warning Scheme in 1982 (Helliwell, 1985), not only to identify the sick doctor, but to assist his or her safe return to work. In addition, in the same year a Department of Health guidance circular was issued setting out the procedures to be adopted if such a case became known to the colleagues of the doctor concerned. While the intention is obviously to protect patients as far as possible, the procedures were also designed to provide rapid help to these practitioners in need. If assistance could be given at an early stage the doctor could be treated as a sick person, and not as a criminal, which would be the outcome if the abuse were discovered later by others, or brought to light as a consequence of an anaesthetic or other tragedy. Each district health authority was required to set up a committee of senior members of the medical or dental profession to advise and take action on any reported addiction or indeed other incapacity due to illness, if harm to a patient is likely to ensue. This panel is popularly known as the 'Three Wise Men'; it is more correctly the panel set up in accordance with the circular 'Prevention of Harm to Patients Resulting from Physical or Mental Disability of Hospital or Community Medical or Dental Staff' (National Health Service, 1982). As the title implies, it is concerned with health factors as well as addiction.

# References

Association of Anaesthetists of Great Britain and Ireland (1975) Advice to Members from the Council: pollution of the atmosphere of operating theatres. *Anaesthesia*, **30**, 697–699

138    Standards of Care in Anaesthesia

British Medical Association (1990) *A Code of Practice on the Safe Use and Disposal of Sharps* (ed. D. Morgan), British Medical Journal, London

Bruce, D. L., Back, M. J. and Arbit, J. (1974) Trace anaesthetic effects on perceptual cognitive and motor skills, *Anesthesiology*, **40**, 453–458

BS 6834;1987 Active anaesthetic gas scavenging systems. British Standards Institution, London

Buring, J. E., Hennekens, C. H., Magrent, S. L., Rosner, B., Greenberg, E. R. and Colton, T. (1985) Health experiences of operating personnel. *Anesthesiology*, **63**, 325–330

Cohen, E. N., Brown, B. W., Bruce, D. L., Cascorbi, H. F., Corbett, T. H., Jones, T. W. and Whitcher, C. E. (1974) Occupational disease among operating room personnel: a national study. *Anesthesiology*, **41**, 321–340

Department of Health (1990) Heads of Agreement. Ministerial Group on Junior Doctor's Hours, DoH, London

Department of Health and Social Security (1983) *Ventilation of Operating Departments. A Design Guide.* Inter-Authority Working Group 10, DHSS Engineering Data, DoH, London

Editorial (1984) Needlestick transmission of HTVL-iii from a patient infected in Africa. *Lancet*, **2**, 1376–1377

Firth-Cozens, J. (1989) Stress in medical undergraduates and house-officers. *British Journal of Hospital Medicine*, **41**, 161–164

Green, R. A. (1986) Editorial: A matter of vigilance. *Anaesthesia*, **41**, 129–130

Harrison, C. A., Rogers, D. W. and Rosen, M. (1990) Blood contamination of anaesthetic and related staff. *Anaesthesia*, **45**, 831–833

Hawkins, M. R., Vichick, M. D., Silsby, H. D., Kruzich, D. J. and Butler, R. (1985) Sleep and nutritional deprivation and the performance of house-officers. *Journal of Medical Education*, **60**, 530–535

Helliwell, P. J. (1985) Editorial: Helping the sick doctor. *Anaesthesia*, **40**, 221–222

Layzer, R. B., Fishman, R. A. and Schafter, J. A. (1978) Neuropathy following abuse of nitrous oxide. *Neurology*, **28**, 504–506

Linde, H. W. and Bruce, D. L. (1969) Occupational exposure of anesthetists to halothane, nitrous oxide and radiation. *Anesthesiology*, **30**, 363–372

Lowbury, E. J. L., Aycliffe, G. A. J., Geddes, A. M. and Williams, J. D. (1981) *Control of Hospital Infection*, 2nd edn, Chapman and Hall, London

Mazze, R. I. (1985) Editorial: The health hazard of operating room personnel. *Anesthesiology*, **63**, 226–228

National Health Service (1982) *Prevention of Harm to Patients Resulting from Physical or Mental Disability of Hospital or Community Dental Staff*, DHSS Health Circular HC(82), 13 July 1982

Nielsen, H., Vasegaard, M. and Stokes, D. B. (1978) Bacterial contamination of anaesthetic gases. *British Journal of Anaesthesia*, **50**, 811–814

NIOSH (National Institute for Occupational Safety and Health) (1977) *Criteria for a Recommended Standard: Occupational Exposure to Waste Anesthetic Gases and Vapours.* Department of Health, Education, and Welfare publication No. 77-140, US Government Printing Office, Washington, DC

Nunn, J. F., Sharer, N. M. and Gorschein, A. (1982) Megaloblastic haemopoesis after multiple short term exposures to nitrous oxide. *Lancet*, **1**, 1379–1381

Pharoah, P. O. D., Alberman, E., Doyle, P. and Chamberlain, G. (1977) Outcome of pregnancy among women in anaesthetic practice. *Lancet*, **1**, 34–36

Roger, P. L., Lantz, H. C., Henderson, D. K., Parillo, J. and Masur, H. (1989) Admission of AIDS patients to a medical intensive care unit. Cause and outcome. *Critical Care Medicine*, **17**, 113–117

Royal College of Surgeons of England (1990) *A Statement by the College on AIDS and HIV infection*, RCS, London

Salo, M. and Vapaavuormi, M. (1976) Peripheral blood T- and B-lymphocytes in operating theatre personnel. *British Journal of Anaesthesia*, **48**, 877–880

Spence, A. A. (1987) Environmental pollution by inhalational agents. *British Journal of Anaesthesia*, **59**, 96–103

Spence, A. A., Wall, R. A. and Nunn, J. F. (1989) Environmental safety of the anaesthetist. In: *General Anaesthesia* (eds. J. F. Nunn, J. E. Utting and B. R. Brown), 5th edn, Butterworths, London, Chapter 47, p. 598

Stock, J. G. and Strunin, L. (1985) Unexplained hepatitis following halothane. *Anesthesiology*, **63**, 424–439, at page 427

Sweeney, B., Bingham, R. M., Amos, R. J., Petty, A. C. and Cole, Z. P. V. (1985) Toxicity of bone marrow in dentists exposed to nitrous oxide. *British Medical Journal*, **291**, 567–569

Tannenbaum, T. W. and Goldberg, R. J. (1985) Exposure to anaesthetic gases and reproductive outcome. A review of the epidemiological literature. *Journal of Occupational Medicine*, **27**, 659–668

Tedder, R. S. (1983) Towards the control of hepatitis B in hospitals. In: *Recent Advances in Clinical Virology* (ed. A. P. Waterson), Churchill Livingstone, Edinburgh, pp. 217–236

Vessey, M. P. and Nunn, J. F. (1980) Occupational hazards of anaesthesia. *British Medical Journal*, **281**, 696–698

Wallace-Barnhill, G. I., Florez, G., Tarndorf, H. and Craythorne, N. W. B. (1983) The effect of 24 hour duty on the performance of the anesthesiology resident on vigilance, mood and memory tasks. *Anesthesiology*, **59**, A460

Ward, C. S. (1985) Atmospheric pollution. In: *Anaesthetic Equipment*, Baillière Tindall, London, Chapter 15, pp. 272–287

Wyon, D., Lidwell, O. M. and Williams, R. E. O. (1968) Thermal comfort during surgical operations. *Journal of Hygiene*, **66**, 229–248

# 7

# Care in the recovery period

## Definition of the recovery period

It is difficult to define the period of recovery from anaesthesia, for it occurs concurrently with the process of recovery from the surgical or manipulative procedure for which the anaesthetic was administered. From the patient's point of view the definition of recovery may involve an even longer time scale, since he or she may have recovered from the acute effects of the drugs given and be able to respond to stimuli and even enter into a conversation, but the after effects may render the patient amnesic so that the responses are forgotten the next day. Other sequelae of the anaesthetic may remain for many days. The occurrence of certain complications will clearly prolong the recovery time.

The immediate recovery period is the time taken by the patient to be aware of his surroundings and be able to maintain his own protective reflexes, and in most circumstances this is under the supervision of an anaesthetist. It is by any standard a very short time compared to the total convalescent time required for complete recovery from an operation. Farman in 1978 reported an average waking time of $8\frac{1}{2}$ minutes, although the time may be considerably longer, especially after major procedures and in those patients who have received muscle relaxants. The importance of 'recovery time' is that it represents the minimum period before a patient can possibly be discharged from the recovery room. In practice full recovery takes much longer, and postoperative patients are peculiarly vulnerable for some days after surgery. Indeed the modern approach should be for such a patient to move into a system of 'progressive patient care' according to the individual requirements of that patient and the nature of the operation undergone.

Thus the ill-defined end to the process of recovery from surgery and anaesthesia makes the definition of recovery time difficult. For practical purposes it seems to be sensible to divide the process of recovery into two phases, the early period when the patient is at risk because of absence or depression of protective reflexes, and later the more prolonged phase of complete recovery from the drugs. The duration of this phase is obscured by the concomitant recovery from the surgical procedure, and by the use of further drugs, for example analgesics, administered in the postoperative treatment. Cotter (1987) has used the term 'primary recovery period' for that part of recovery before the patient can be safely returned to a normal surgical ward. When the patient is transferred to a general surgical ward the high level of care on a one-to-one basis is no longer required, for the patient is aware and can maintain his own airway, with protective reflexes active, is able to breathe adequately and has a stable circulation. In most hospitals the medical care of the patient in the primary recovery period has become the responsibility of the anaesthetist, although the minute-to-minute supervision is delegated to specially trained nurses. This recovery should take place in a fully equipped and staffed recovery room, in close proximity to the operating theatre. In the absence of such a facility supervision of the patient in this stage of treatment becomes the sole responsibility of the anaesthetist who administered the anaesthetic, and cannot, in the opinion of the authors, be safely delegated.

## Adverse events in the primary recovery period

From the available evidence it is possible to predict that between 5 and 10% of patients, after undergoing surgery, will experience unanticipated and undesirable events that will require intervention, sometimes urgently. The five events which occur commonly are hypotension, hypertension, arrhythmias, hypovolaemia and the various airway problems. These are not specifically related to the anaesthetic agents used. There are also some residual effects due to the continuing effects of drugs commonly employed in anaesthesia, for example paralysis can persist following the use of neuromuscular blocking agents and is not infrequently seen after the use of atracurium and vecuronium if reversal is attempted too soon after the administration of the last dose. Patients easily become hypoxic, and although the ventilatory depression may be due to the lingering effects of the general anaesthetic, it is more likely to be seen if an excessive dose of opioid analgesic has been given during the operation, or in the recovery room afterwards (Beard, Jick and Walker, 1986). Improving circulation may release opioids from the site of a previous intramuscular injection. Lastly, it should always be remembered that any patient with depressed reflexes is in danger of aspirating gastric contents, and because of this the airway should be safeguarded by posture if this is compatible with the overall care of the patient. This is especially important in the young and the old.

142 Standards of Care in Anaesthesia

Cooper, Leigh and Tring (1989) studied the anaesthetic and surgical history of patients admitted to the Intensive Care Unit (ICU) of a district general hospital because of complications of the anaesthetic technique. Over a 5-year period 81 780 patients received a general or local anaesthetic, or intravenous sedation and one patient in 1543 – 53 patients in all – had to be admitted to the unit as a result. These represented 2% of the admissions to the unit with a mortality rate of 17%. In 26% of the admissions it was thought that the complications could have been avoided. Of the 53 admissions, the majority of the precipitating events occurred in the recovery period, that is in 33 patients. Of these patients 24 suffered ventilatory failure, five aspiration of gastric contents, two respiratory obstruction, and the remaining two had acute pulmonary oedema and a hydrothorax following the insertion of a central venous line from the antecubital fossa respectively. In this subgroup the authors thought that avoidable factors were present in six of these cases. The largest group of admissions, 24 in all, were patients with ventilatory failure after attempted reversal of nondepolarizing neuromuscular blocking agents. This group had the high average age of 70, and were equally divided between elective (11) and emergency (13) surgery. From the detailed figures, the authors conclude that elective postoperative ventilation should be given to elderly patients undergoing emergency laparotomy. Similar results were reported in the survey of Barnes and Havill in 1980, although their admission rate was double that of the later study, for a similar number of procedures.

# Hypoxaemia in the recovery period

Hypoxaemia is a serious hazard in the primary recovery period, and would afflict, to a greater or lesser degree, all patients if they did not receive supplemental oxygen. Hypoxaemia following surgery can always be found in patients breathing air, and although it may persist only a few minutes after a very short anaesthetic, it may be present for days in more major operations, especially those on the thorax and upper abdomen. This was shown by Palmer and Gardiner in 1964 in relation to patients undergoing partial gastrectomy.

Postoperative hypoxaemia has two principal causes: the first is the continuation of the factors that reduce respiratory efficiency during anaesthesia. Reduced tone in the chest wall musculature together with alterations in vascular and bronchomotor tone persist after the anaesthetic, and this may continue for some days. In addition, there is impairment of the control of breathing, which results in episodic obstructive apnoea, and which is exacerbated by opioids (Jones, Sapford and Wheatley, 1990). The lateral position adopted as a 'safe posture' can also impair the efficiency of the lower lung. The patients have a significant shunt within the lung from right to left, reducing the arterial $Pao_2$ by 3–4 kPa, which may be worsened by areas of mismatch between perfusion and ventilation. Hypoventilation may also be present as a result of the drugs used in the anaesthetic or because of postoperative pain. Obstructive apnoea can be induced by opioids and hypoxaemia can be related to the sleep often associated with their administration. A low cardiac output, shivering and old age may exacerbate the problem.

Craig (1981) thought that the early postoperative hypoxaemia was largely due to the anaesthetic and the agents used, and the later hypoxaemia was due to opioids. It has been suggested that post-operative hypoxaemia, if allowed to persist, may be associated with a higher incidence of myocardial ischaemia and infarction.

Thus all postoperative patients should receive supplemental oxygen, and it may be necessary to continue this after the primary recovery period, even for some days, when the patient has been returned to a surgical ward. Oxygen can be delivered by a face mask with a regulated gas flow. Smith, Canning and Crul (1989) have shown that this can be effectively monitored by using a pulse oximeter, with a lower alarm limit set at 90%, provided the patient is not cold and is in a stable cardiovascular condition, with a mean blood pressure over 50 mmHg. The simple method of adding oxygen will restore the arterial oxygen levels in most cases unless the intrapulmonary shunt is large. If the immediate postoperative hypoxaemia is not rapidly relieved the patient should be intubated and mechanical ventilation instituted with intermittent positive pressure ventilation and possibly a high end-expiratory pressure. The use of continuous positive airway pressure masks is not recommended even in that group of patients who have adequate carbon dioxide elimination in the presence of hypoxaemia.

It is essential that recovery rooms should not only be equipped with pulse oximeters to measure oxygen saturation but also have available the means to analyse an arterial oxygen sample.

## The primary recovery period

The recovery of a patient from the effects of the anaesthetic begins in the operating theatre as the anaesthetic drugs are reversed or withdrawn, and the conduct of this phase of care should be under the direct supervision of the anaesthetist. It is important that the safety of the patient should not be compromised by the apparent confusion that often follows the completion of one operation and the start of the next. In particular the individual designated as the assistant to the anaesthetist, whether a nurse or an Operating Department Assistant (ODA), should be available exclusively to help with the initial recovery phase and the transfer to the recovery room. Transfer should not be effected until the patient is in a stable condition, is properly oxygenated and in a safe posture after the removal of the airway or endotracheal tube. On some occasions the endotracheal tube will be left in place, and finally removed in the recovery room. All the staff present in the operating theatre, and this most certainly includes the surgeons, should remember that at this time the patient will gradually become aware of his or her surroundings, and most importantly, that hearing is the first faculty to recover. Injudicious chatter at this time can be most harmful, and can even suggest to the patient that the operation is not yet complete, and therefore he or she has become aware during the operation.

The transfer of the patient and the handing over of care to the trained recovery nurses should be done by the anaesthetist, for the task is too important to delegate. Once in the recovery room, the aims should be clear. These are to allow safe recovery of all airway reflexes and muscle power, to prevent hypoxaemia from whatever cause, to note quickly and then, if necessary, to treat effectively alterations in blood pressure, and to note the onset of cardiac arrhythmias. The patient should be made comfortable by all forms of nursing care, and any analgesia required should be given promptly. It is important that the effects of the first dose of postoperative analgesia should be noted and fully charted, especially any untoward effect on the respiratory pattern and oxygenation. Proper charts should be kept of the blood and fluids lost, and of the amounts of fluid transfused. It will also be necessary to care for sites of the infusions and the cannulae employed for invasive monitoring. Finally the staff must be aware of the possible complications that may occur in relation to the surgical and anaes-thetic procedure undergone, and be able to recognize and treat them correctly at an early stage. It goes without saying that to perform these duties effectively the staff must be well trained, be present with their patients on a one-to-one basis, certainly in the early stages of recovery, be able to call on other nursing assistance and finally have rapid access to skilled anaesthetic help by means of an alarm call system.

# Recovery room facilities

## Historical background

In the majority of operating theatre complexes within the United Kingdom it is difficult to conceive the conditions that existed before the introduction of 'postoperative observation rooms' or recovery wards in 1955 (Jolly and Lee, 1957). No routine list should now be undertaken without this facility and indeed the need is recognized by the Department of Heath (1967). The College of Anaesthetists, then the Faculty, in its training requirements cites the need for adequate recovery facilities to be available 24 hours a day, before recognizing a training post (Faculty of Anaesthetists, 1987). The Association of Anaesthetists of Great Britian and Ireland (1985) have published standards for recovery facilities. In the United States recovery rooms have to be provided (US Department of Health, Education, and Welfare 1978).

Goodchild (1988) found in a survey of three hospital regions in the United Kingdom that the clinical work had not altered materially since the inception of recovery rooms, for they are still dominated by cardiovascular and respiratory problems, especially upper airway obstruction. The survey found, however, that 70% of hospitals simply do not provide facilities and staffing levels which meet the requirements of the Association of Anaesthetists, and two-thirds of those hospitals which had recovery rooms provided no service out of routine hours for emergency work. Particular defects were the deficient staffing ratios and poor level of monitoring and other equipment. These findings are confirmed by the survey on mortality associated with anaesthesia reported by Lunn and Mushin (1982), which showed that one-third of the patients who died within six days of operation did not receive care in adequate recovery facilities.

In an ideal system the hospital services would be organized for a continuous flow of patients from theatres to the recovery area, and from there either to an Intensive Therapy Unit, if needed, or to an area of high dependency care. The time spent in each of these phases before return to a normal ward would depend on the procedures undergone.

It would seem, then, that much improvement in the facilities so far provided is required to achieve optimum patient care, and any improvement will involve considerable expenditure. Nevertheless, anaesthetists as individuals and as a body must not be persuaded by hospital authorities to continue to work in the absence of proper facilities. It is probable that with the inception of National Health Service Indemnity the hospital authorities will seek to minimize the legal costs and damages incurred by the tragic errors that can be ascribed to poor provision of recovery areas, and may find expenditure on preventative measures well worth while. The facilities that should be provided for the period of primary recovery will now be described.

## Site

The recovery room must be adjacent to the operating theatre suite in which the operation is performed. To transfer a patient a long distance immediately after operation really negates the whole concept of this facility. If this is geographically or organizationally impossible then sufficient staff and monitoring apparatus should be provided for the transfer, but the organizers of such a system must realize the additional risk to the patient that exists. Thus it can be seen that at least for the provision of anaesthetic and recovery facilities, the concept of a single theatre associated with a ward for a particular specialty is less than ideal, for staff and equipment costs will limit the standard of service that can be provided. Those working in such an area will be deprived of the support and assistance that a bigger unit can provide. This also applies to all but the largest obstetric units.

It is also essential that any recovery area is not isolated from the main hospital, so that communication can be continuous with the ward staff, and the transfer back to the surgical ward can be easily accomplished. Ideally the Intensive Care Unit (ICU) and high dependency beds should also be nearby.

## Staff

In the United Kingdom the number of recovery beds required is assessed as three for every operating theatre, more if the intensive care facilities are inadequate. This could be insufficient where the theatre being served has a list of minor cases with a rapid turnover, for the recovery of these patients is every bit as important as in the major procedure, and requires a considerable amount of observation and charting. Although the nurses may be controlled from an ICU, the staffing of these two areas should be separate. The recovery room should be open at any time the theatres it serves are in use. As the survey of Goodchild showed, this last condition is not always met in the United Kingdom, despite the stated training requirements of the College of Anaesthetists.

The status of the nursing staff is vital, for the recovery room must be staffed by experienced, trained nurses with one in overall charge on all shifts. Each patient needs the services of one nurse continuously during the primary recovery phase, and there must be additional 'runners' as required. When consciousness returns it is usually assumed that a nurse can supervise more patients, perhaps up to three, and still be available to assist others. The nurse in charge must watch carefully to prevent the ratio of staff to patients falling below a safety level, because the recovery area must maintain enough 'free' nurses to provide for the emergency situation. Nursing trainees should be supernumerary, and never left in charge of a patient on their own. If the one-to-one relationship of nurse to patient cannot be maintained no further patients should be admitted and the operating lists temporarily suspended until the overcrowding is relieved, or a decision is made to allow subsequent patients to recover in the operating theatre under the supervision of the anaesthetist.

Although each anaesthetist assumes responsibility for his or her own patients while in the recovery room, one member of the department must be nominated to assume the responsibility for the protocols and to liaise with the sister-in-charge to assist with the protocols and training. This person will obviously have a part to play in supervising the purchase and use of ventilating and monitoring equipment. A further vital part of this person's role is to ensure that all the anaesthetists and surgeons comply with the necessary rules applying to the recovery room.

## Equipment

Each bay should be well illuminated with light equivalent to normal daylight, have access to electrical power points and be equipped with fixed points for oxygen and suction. A compressed air source, although not essential is convenient for driving ventilators if required. An adequate working surface should be provided. It is essential that the beds or trolleys are not too crowded, so that work on each patient may proceed unimpeded. It is vital that the beds and trolleys used can be tipped either head- or foot-down by means of a simple lever action, and not require physical lifting, and they should be provided with side rails to prevent restless patients falling out. The bays should have a convenient store for suckers of all types, airways and oxygen masks. A means of inflating the lungs of a patient should always be on hand, together with intubation equipment and a full range of endotracheal tube introducers and bougies, although not necessarily in each bay.

The recovery room should also have the instruments for minor procedures and wound care. More important are those required for emergency intubation, including bronchoscopes of all types and sizes, and the means to perform a tracheostomy. The usual paraphernalia associated with the treatment of a cardiorespiratory arrest is essential. It is desirable that each bay has an alarm to summon the hospital cardiac arrest team.

Many units now have the apparatus for basic 'laboratory' investigations to be performed on site. This means that the syringes and other equipment needed should be readily available. Due care must be exercised in the interpretation of these tests, as the stringent controls associated with a main hospital laboratory are lacking.

As X-rays are commonly needed in the area, there should be a large viewing screen available. Frequently these films are taken with a portable X-ray machine as an emergency after the patient has been admitted. This work is seriously hampered if the bays are too small.

Lastly, in addition to normal telephones, there must be the means of summoning urgent medical and other assistance. Thus as well as the cardiac arrest bell there should be an alarm bell which sounds in the theatre area. The theatre staff, both medical and nursing, must be familiar with this sound and respond to it immediately unless absolutely committed themselves. Adequate provision must be made for those times when the staffing levels are low, such as night time and weekends.

## Drugs

The recovery room must hold an adequate supply of the drugs that may be required. In a unit engaged with patients from all types of surgery this means an extensive stock, but those drugs commonly used will be well known to both medical and nursing staff. The less well known are usually needed quickly and so must be on site in small initial supply, and the whereabouts of the main stock known.

In addition, there must be a supply of the commonly used intravenous fluids and blood products. A means of pressurizing the bags or bottles of fluid must be available in case a rapid transfusion is required. It is desirable that the transfusion can be brought to the right temperature by means of a blood warmer when fluid is given rapidly.

# Failure to meet standards

## Inadequate facilities

As has been suggested in the previous section, a dangerous situation arises when inadequate facilities are dignified with the name of a recovery room. Examples of mishaps which have arisen because of the lack of adequate facilities are common throughout the world, especially in the files of the Defence Organizations; for example, the use of a recovery 'bay' in the theatre corridor, provided with minimum facilities, and with no proper staff designated and not fully equipped with the necessary apparatus.

The provision of a suitable recovery room is the responsibility of the hospital, but an anaesthetist undertaking to provide an anaesthetic service must satisfy himself that the care provided is of a sufficient standard, or perform the task of supervising the primary recovery period himself. This is, of course, safe, but will not allow a rapid turnover of cases. In the absence of a proper recovery room this must be done in the theatre itself, until the primary recovery phase is complete. This means that a single-handed practitioner will be unable to start the next case on an operating list until this phase is complete and it is safe to hand the patient over to the care of the surgical ward staff.

## *Inadequate staff*

The nurses who look after the postoperative patients must be trained in the special skills required and be in sufficient numbers properly to discharge their duties. When a recovery room is first set up a precise standard of care and the level of staffing must be agreed between the users, that is the anaesthetists and surgeons, and the nursing administration. The staff ratio used must be one-to-one for unconscious patients with a minimum of one person free of immediate duties to act as runner or assistant. This means that even if there is only one patient, two nurses are required.

It is now expected that this staffing should be available throughout the 24 hours of the day. It is to be regretted that this standard is not yet universal in the United Kingdom, despite the efforts of the College of Anaesthetists, who will not recognize hospitals for training purposes in the absence of this facility. Although many anaesthetists, often of junior status, work without this service, it is now probably an unacceptable standard of care. It is possible that in the near future anaesthetic departments serving hospitals without full out-of-hours service should decline to run an emergency service. No consultant should allow such a deficient service to be the norm for the junior anaesthetist in training, working alone to provide out-of-hours emergency cover.

Likewise the anaesthetist must appreciate the problems which arise at times even in the best staffed and run units. When the nurse in charge of a recovery room has in his or her care the full number of patients for whom staff are available, then admissions should temporarily cease. This decision is for the nursing staff alone, possibly in consultation with the nominated anaesthetist. It should not be overridden by others. The immediate care of the patient then reverts to the anaesthetist. It should not be left to an untrained nurse in the theatres.

# Emergency drills

Even in the best regulated environment, untoward events occur, and the recovery room is not free of them. The most serious emergencies that occur are cardiovascular collapse and respiratory obstruction or failure. All the staff should be rehearsed in correct treatment of these situations and the part they are to play in the emergency situation. This must not be left until the crisis happens. The other vital factor at these times is the ease of communication with other parts of the hospital to call assistance, especially the cardiac arrest team.

# Recovery room procedures

## *Charts and communications*

The provision of a recovery ward does not permit an anaesthetist to abrogate responsibility for an unconscious patient entirely. The person who renders a patient unconscious and thus without the normal protective reflexes must undertake the responsibility of caring for that patient until the patient is able to do so himself. This overriding responsibility can be properly delegated to another anaesthetist at any time after induction, provided the handover between the two is adequate to ensure a full knowledge of preceding events.

At the end of the operative procedure delegation will be to a nurse who has received a proper training in recovery room procedures and is familiar with the protocols of the hospital. The anaesthetist should be satisfied at that point that the patient is well enough to be passed into the care of a nurse; that is to say, that the anaesthetist expects the patient to proceed to a normal recovery without foreseeable complications and that the recovery room and its staffing are adequate. Clearly at this time the patient must be lying in a safe position, the degree of sedation must be lightening, with normal respiration and with the circulatory parameters stable. The nurse must be able to give the patient undivided attention for the succeeding minutes until the primary recovery has occurred, and must be fully informed of the patient's condition and be familiar with the protocols of the unit concerned. Despite these provisions the anaesthetist must be available within a few minutes' call of the recovery room until the patient is fully awake and in a stable condition. It is reasonable for the anaesthetist to hand over this responsibility to a suitable colleague who is available near the unit, perhaps by handing over to a 'duty' colleague. It is quite unacceptable to leave an unconscious patient in nursing care with no rapid access to skilled medical help.

The conclusion to be drawn from the account given above is that there is no specific time limit on the continuing task of the anaesthetist to care for a patient. It is not justifiable to leave unconscious patients in the sole care of a nurse after an anaesthetic. In those patients where recovery is prolonged the anaesthetist may have to be present for an extended period. The anaesthetist should not leave the patient in the care of the recovery room nursing staff until all the relevant details of the surgical procedure, the anaesthetic technique and any important history of the patient or of complications have been communicated to the recovery staff. The intraoperative anaesthetic chart should be available, and some guidance given on the requirements for special observations in the particular case.

During the stay in the recovery room, all relevant findings must be recorded, and those notes handed on to the staff who next care for the patient, whether they are surgical ward staff or the ICU staff. The chart should be understood by those taking over and also be compatible with other hospital notes. This is especially important when recording the drugs given and the time of their administration, and when the blood loss and the fluid replacement is being charted. The ward should also be aware of the names of the medical staff involved in the case and their immediate movements. Patient transfers should not occur until the receiving ward is sufficiently staffed to cope with the returning patient.

Communication is especially important where the patient has a continuing regional blockade, intended for postoperative pain relief. The most important fact to be imparted in these circumstances is the name of the doctor to be called if the need arises.

## Monitoring

The primary 'monitor' employed in the recovery room is the clinical observations of a properly trained nurse. This also ensures the presence by the bedside of the nurse during the period of primary recovery. The common clinical parameters are measured very frequently at first, but gradually settle to a regular pattern. The pulse rate, blood pressure and respiratory rate, together with the temperature in certain cases, are the minimum observations required. For these a visible clock with a second hand, a thermometer and a sphygmomanometer are required. Fluid input and output should also be charted, together with any apparent blood loss.

The basic observations can be supplemented by many monitors. The most useful, especially when non-white patients and children are involved, is a pulse oximeter. Self-recording noninvasive blood pressure apparatus and the electrocardiogram are important. There should be facilities for direct arterial pressure measurement and the analysis of an arterial blood sample for blood gases.

## Specific management

There are a number of problems that should be the special concern of the recovery room staff. It is usual for the patients to arrive in the area on their sides, to protect the airway form regurgitation. In many cases this posture can be maintained until the patient is awake. This position is also safe and helps preserve the unintubated airway. The patient should be receiving oxygen through a face mask. The observation of the patency of the airway and the preservation of adequate oxygenation must be the first task of the recovery nurse.

It is not uncommon for patients to feel nauseated or even vomit after anaesthesia, and this can be largely controlled by the use of suitable antiemetic drugs. These are better given prophylactically by the anaesthetist at the end of the operation, but the effects must be noted and further drugs given if indicated. Likewise, the nurse in the recovery area has a key role in ensuring that the patient receives adequate analgesic drugs, and that the effects of these drugs are noted before the return to the surgical ward. The surgical ward staff should be informed by the recovery room nurses of the dose and time of administration of the analgesics and antiemetics, including those given in the theatre by the anaesthetist.

In hospitals in the United Kingdom it has been the custom to write the prescription for postoperative analgesic and anti-emetic drugs 'as required' ('prn'). In most institutions this instruction means, in the absence of an added time limit by the prescriber, that the drug can be repeated 4 hours after the last dose, if the patient's condition warrants it. This requirement includes any premedication dose and that given in the course of the operation. This precaution is essential to prevent overdosage of these depressant drugs. The responsible anaesthetist must include clear instructions on this matter, bearing in mind that in the immediate aftermath of an operation a shorter interval may be desirable. It is fortunate that the use of syringe pumps and continuous infusions, together with regional analgesia or epidural opioids, have improved the quality of postoperative pain management, providing more effective management without the use of large intramuscular doses of analgesics.

It must be admitted that the management of postoperative pain is not optimal in this country, compared with some institutions in the United States of America, perhaps because it is often left to the most junior hospital staff with little supervision. Many patients are subjected to needless distress by unrelieved pain and discomfort after operations. Because of their concern over the lack of progress in the management of postoperative pain, the Royal College of Surgeons of England set up a working party to consider all aspects of postoperative pain relief, with the assistance of many others, including anaesthetists. The report concludes that an Acute Pain Service should be introduced in all major hospitals performing surgery in the United Kingdom (Commission on the Provision of Surgical Services, 1990).

Agitated patients are sometimes seen in the recovery room. There are many causes of postoperative agitation, but it is a feature of patients who are hypoxic without cyanosis, and if seen should lead all concerned to investigate this possibility as a priority. It may be associated with incomplete reversal of the longer-acting neuromuscular blocking agents. Clinical tests of the successful reversal of blockade, such as hand grip and lifting the head from the pillow, can be supplemented by specific tests of function using a peripheral nerve stimulator (Viby-Morgensen, Jorgensen and Ording, 1979). Other causes of agitation include the presence of pain, a full bladder or a urinary catheter, hypercapnoea, uncomfortable postures in bed and the receding effects of the other anaesthetic agents. It is also produced by the use of sedative premedicant drugs without appropriate analgesics. This can often be seen in children given phenothiazines and barbiturates, and in older patients, with hyoscine.

Shivering also occurs in the recovering patient. This can be a manifestation of heat loss during surgery, resulting in hypothermia, but has also been described following the administration of volatile agents, especially halothane. It occurs more commonly in young muscular individuals, and can lead to a greatly increased oxygen demand. Although the use of these agents may result in some heat loss due to the peripheral vasodilation, there is some evidence of loss of central control of spinal reflexes and thus of muscular activity after the volatile agents have been used (Hammel, 1988; Sessler et al., 1988).

Impairment of mental responses occurs after surgery and anaesthesia, but apparently recovers rapidly subsequently. Korttila has studied this impairment of cognitive and psychomotor function extensively (Korttila, 1986). Mental impairment may occur after anaesthesia, especially in the elderly. Minimal short-term mental impairment occurs for up to 7 days even in young patients, but in some the impairment is exacerbated and leads to a persistent change (Smith, 1991). At the other end of the age scale, anaesthesia can have adverse psychological effects on children and takes the form of bad dreams and social withdrawal in the short term, but may lead to behavioural changes that may require psychiatric treatment (Meursing, 1989).

## Discharge from the recovery room

No patient should be discharged from a recovery area unless several problems have been correctly dealt with. The first is that satisfactory analgesia is established and any unpleasant symptoms, such as nausea, have been treated. Although these symptoms are often a direct result of the surgery, they are treated by the anaesthetist. Before discharge to the ward the other surgical aspects of the patient's care must be checked to exclude the need for urgent return to the theatre. Haemorrhage is clearly the major problem here. The wound dressings and any wound drains should be inspected and all prescribed drugs should have been given and the patient's reaction to them monitored.

Any attempts to discharge a patient from a recovery area prematurely when these conditions have not been satisfied nullifies the benefits to the patient and wastes the costs of providing such an area. It leads to a false sense of security by the surgeon, anaesthetist and nursing staff alike.

There are some patients who have a prolonged recovery time. The cause of this may be suspected by the anaesthetist, but many cases arise with no predisposing cause. These patients require full supervision for some hours after surgery, and should properly be admitted to a high dependency unit or ICU.

## Recovery after day care surgery

After day care surgery under general anaesthesia or regional blockade, patients are kept under observation in a recovery area for a period until fit to return home. The problems of the recovery period after day care surgery are not fundamentally different from those relating to inpatients. Because the patient is returning home, those in charge of the unit will have to be quite satisfied that the patient is sufficiently recovered from the procedure to be allowed home in the care of relatives or friends, who though loving and caring, may be quite unsophisticated and unskilled in medical matters. It is therefore important to ensure in so far as possible that there are no untoward effects. Before discharge, the patient must be able to look after him- or herself without assistance, even though the return home must be accompanied by an adult, the alternative being an ambulance if there is no suitable person to act as escort or if the journey by public transport is too arduous. Preferably the patient should not be left alone for the subsequent 24 hours.

The decision to discharge is frequently taken by the nursing staff, following protocols laid down for the unit, although an anaesthetist or surgeon must also be available to assist with difficult cases. There are many quantitative tests suggested to ensure that a patient is fit for discharge, many involving the use of a pencil and paper by the patient, but none is simple enough, with unequivocal results, to be used every day. The practical decision is best made by an experienced nurse on clinical grounds (Cooper, 1987). This decision will be based on the patient's ability to walk steadily unaided and the normal response in conversation. These positive findings together with the restrictions placed on the patient's activities in the next 24–48 hours should suffice.

It may be safer to base the discharge from a day care unit on a precise scoring system, somewhat similar to the scoring system used for the newborn with the 'Apgar' score (Apgar, 1953). If such a system is used in place of the nurse's clinical judgement, it must give consistent results and be simple to use. Steward (1975) devised such a system, omitting factors such as colour and blood pressure, the first because it was difficult to quantify, and the second because it has little relevance to wakefulness. The three factors examined to calculate the score are: consciousness, the airway and movement. Patients who are still unresponsive score 0, responding patients 1 and those fully awake 2. With regard to the airway, those not maintaining an airway score 0, those maintaining an airway score 1 and those who cough on command 2. In a similar way movement scores 0, 1 or 2 from not moving, through nonpurposeful movements to purposeful movements. A score of 6 indicates a fully recovered patient, but a lesser number does indicate the progress made by the patient from a base line of zero over a known time course. Robertson, MacGregor and Jones, (1977), when investigating the effects of doxapram in the recovery from outpatient anaesthesia, devised a similar but more cumbersome system.

When discharged, patients should receive written instructions to take away with them, for the spoken word is often not remembered in the unusual situation of the operation and anaesthetic. These instructions would include an injunction not to drive or use dangerous machines for 24 hours, and a note indicating the contact if a complication such as haemorrhage should occur. The specific instruction, given to patients after day care surgery and anaesthesia, not to drink alcohol or take drugs not known to the unit, and not use machinery or drive a motor vehicle until at least 24 hours have passed, are vitally important. The residual effects of the surgical operation and anaesthetic on the patients' concentration and hence their performance may persist for a longer period even than this and at the present time there is no absolutely satisfactory test to measure when a patient has fully recovered from these less obvious effects.

## Late complications associated with anaesthesia

There are few studies of long-term complications of anaesthesia, but when, as is currently the case, there is considerable emphasis on standards and audit these complications need to be evaluated. Duncan and Cohen (1987) recently published the results of a 9-year prospective study. They found the risk of postoperative morbidity is increased with higher ASA physical status and the duration of the anaesthetic. Patients who experience intraoperative complications, or those that have a pure spinal or narcotic-based anaesthetic, also have an increase in postoperative complications. Furthermore, it seems that the incidence of postoperative complications decreases with the increasing experience of the anaesthetist. The two most obvious postoperative events that complicate recovery, or indeed cause death, are myocardial infarction and pulmonary embolus. The anaesthetic management before, during and after the operation influences the outcome in both these cases and indeed, with the latter, prophylaxis with subcutaneous heparin started before surgery improves the outlook.

## Standard of care in surgical and medical wards

The provision of a recovery ward ensures the case of the patient in the primary recovery period, but the need for the anaesthetist to exercise some supervision continues in the general surgical ward. Obviously this must include patients with ongoing regional analgesia, and continuous analgesic infusions. It is also important in certain patients, such as the elderly, who may become confused, and in certain pre-existing medical conditions, where the anaesthetist can be expected to have special expertise in the side effects of surgery and anaesthesia.

It cannot be emphasized too strongly that the medical staff must continue the care and write notes at the required intervals. If there is any reason to suspect an adverse response to the anaesthetic or the drugs and techniques used the anaesthetist should visit and make notes. A postoperative visit does not take long and is important in those cases where regional anaesthesia has been used, and especially if a complication such as post-spinal headache ensues. This condition can be ameliorated with the correct treatment given promptly.

## Continuity of care: transfer to intensive care unit

In many ICUs, although anaesthetists provide the continuing care, the rotas may not include the anaesthetist who was present at the patient's operation. The fact that care is provided in this way does not absolve the original anaesthetist of the case from exhibiting some interest in the continuing care, and even taking it over.

## References

Apgar, V. (1953) A proposal for a new method of evaluation of the newborn infant. *Anesthesia and Analgesia*, **32**, 260–267

Association of Anaesthetists of Great Britain and Ireland (1985) *Post-anaesthetic Recovery Facilities*, London

Barnes, P. J. and Havill, J. H. (1980) Anaesthetic complications requiring intensive care: a five year revue. *Anesthesia and Intensive Care*, **8**, 404–409

Beard, K., Jick, H. and Walker, A. M. (1986) Adverse respiratory events occurring in the recovery room after general anesthesia. *Anesthesiology*, **64**, 269–272

Commission on the Provision of Surgical Services (1990) *Report of the Working Party on Pain after Surgery*, Royal College of Surgeons of England, London

Cooper, A. L., Leigh, J. M. and Tring, I. C. (1989) Admissions to the intensive care unit after complications of anaesthetic technique after ten years: the first five years. *Anaesthesia*, **44**, 953–958

Cooper, G. M. (1987) Day-case anaesthesia. In: *Hazards and Complications of Anaesthesia* (ed. T. H. Taylor and E. Major), Churchill Livingstone, Edinburgh, p. 407

Cotter, J. (1987) Complications of recovery from anaesthesia. In: *Hazards and Complications of Anaesthesia* (ed. T. H. Taylor and E. Major), Churchill Livingstone, Edinburgh

Craig, D. B. (1981) Post-operative recovery of pulmonary function. *Anesthesia and Analgesia*, **60**, 40–52

Department of Health and Social Security (1967) *Hospital Building Recommendations*, C9 SFB, HMSO, London

Duncan, P. G. and Cohen, M. M. (1987) Postoperative complications: factors of significance to anaesthetic practice. *Canadian Journal of Anaesthesia*, **34**, 2–8

Faculty of Anaesthetists of the Royal College of Surgeons of England (1987) *General Professional Training Guide*, London

Farman, J. V. (1978) The work of the recovery room. *British Journal of Hospital Medicine*, **19**, 606–616

Goodchild, C. S. (1988) Post-operative recovery rooms. Staffing and facilities in three regions in the United Kingdom. *Anaesthesia*, **43**, 829–832

Hammel, H. T. (1988) Editorial: Anesthetics and body temperature regulation. *Anesthesiology*, **68**, 833–835

Jolly, C. and Lee, J. A. (1957) Post-operative observation ward. *Anaesthesia*, **12**, 49–52

Jones, J. G., Sapford, D. J. and Wheatley, R. G. (1990) Postoperative hypoxaemia: mechanism and time course. *Anaesthesia*, **45**, 566–573

Korttila, K. (1986) Postanesthetic cognitive and psychomotor impairment. *International Anesthesiology Clinics*, **24**, 59–74

Lunn, J. N. and Mushin, W. W. (1982) *Mortality Associated with Anaesthesia.* Nuffield Provincial Hospitals Trust, London

Meursing, A. E. C. (1989) Psychological effcts of anaesthesia in children. *Current Opinion in Anaesthesiology*, **2**, 335–338

Palmer, K. N. V. and Gardiner, A. J. S. (1964) Effect of partial gastrectomy on pulmonary physiology. *British Medical Journal*, **1**, 347–349

Robertson, G. S., MacGregor, D. M. and Jones, C. J. (1977) Evaluation of doxapram for arousal from general anaesthesia in outpatients. *British Journal of Anaesthesia*, **49**, 133–140

Sessler, D. I., Israel, D., Pozos, R. S., Pozos, M. and Rubinstein, E. H. (1988) Spontaneous post-anaesthetic tremor does not resemble thermoregulatory shivering. *Anesthesiology*, **68**, 843–850

Smith, C. M. (1991) Anaesthesia and mental impairment in the elderly. Personal communication

Smith, D. C., Canning, J. J. and Crul, J. F. (1989) Pulse oximetry in the recovery room. *Anaesthesia*, **44**, 345–348

Steward, D. J. (1975) A simplified scoring system for the post-operative recovery room. *Canadian Anaesthetic Society Journal*, **22**, 111–115

United States Department of Health, Education, and Welfare (1978) *Minimum Requirements for Construction and Equipment for Hospital Medical Facilities*, US Government Printing Office, Washington, DC

Viby-Morgensen, J., Jorgensen, B. C. and Ording, H. (1979) Residual curarisation in the recovery room. *Anesthesiology*, **50**, 539–541

# 8

# Standards and audit

The British National Health Service (NHS) Review White Paper (Working for Patients, 1989) defines medical audit as the systematic, critical analysis of the quality of medical care, including the procedures used for diagnosis and treatment, the use of resources, and the resulting outcome and quality of life for the patient. Quality assurance is the process in which the provision and performance of care is measured against expectations or standards so that the information thus gained is used to improve the delivery of care. Medical audit is thus an essential component in quality assurance. Risk management is primarily focused on lessening the risk of litigation. Clinical risk management is one of the aims of quality assurance in which clinical practice is reviewed and recommendations made to minimize the incidence of, and undesirable outcome from, events that chiefly adversely affect patients, but may also have an impact on staff or visitors to hospital.

To perform this process a task is identified, and in clinical anaesthesia this will include preventing avoidable morbidity and mortality. Information on the relevant practice of anaesthesia is then collected and, if the results indicate the need, steps are taken to improve the results of treatment by altering practice. The process does not end there but must continue with further audit to assess the result of the changes (Brown, 1984). Audit is now an integral part of the processes in the National Health Service in which all clinicians are expected to participate (Report of the Standing Medical Advisory Committee, 1990). What to audit, how to audit and why to audit is not always clear, and where the time, resources and manpower to perform the audit are to come from is not yet apparent. We live in a world of limited resources and conflicting calls on those resources. Although the economic consequences of medical audit cannot be ignored, a practising doctor's concern with medical audit should primarily be with patient outcome and the quality of medical care.

Thus it is important to make a process of audit acceptable to busy doctors who have the primary interest of improving patient care. This is more likely if the purpose is, at least in part, educational, i.e. towards improved patient care, if participation is voluntary and if control is by clinical equals. The standards preferably should be set by those responsible for the service, and the method of audit should be interesting and not too time-consuming (Shaw, 1980).

For medical audit to work it is imperative to have a clear idea of the objectives of medical care. A possible formulation for a department of anaesthesia may be as follows:

1. Specify the 'aims' of the anaesthetic department: this will include the administration of so many anaesthetics, the provision of so many epidurals, and care for an estimated number of patients in intensive care, etc.

2. Define the standard of care: this standard needs regular review taking into consideration changes in anaesthetic practice. Examples are no deaths or major morbidity in ASA I and II patients, less than 0.5% inadvertent dural puncture, levels of outcome in intensive care related to severity of patient's illness etc.

3. Maintain accurate records to see if 'aims' and standards are achieved.

4. Hold regular compulsory audit meetings: these should discuss matters such as anaesthetic deaths and complications, out-of-hours work, staffing arrangements and workload. A record should be kept of attendance and of subjects discussed. Decisions should be taken and regular review made of the effect of any changes.

5. An annual review should be undertaken: this should consider the work of the department including the success achieved in reaching the predetermined goals.

Several anaesthetic organizations are specifically interested in preventing anaesthetic-related morbidity and mortality by providing guidance on standards of care and outcome with aspects of clinical practice. The Quality of Practice Committee of the College of Anaesthetists has the remit in the United Kingdom of exploring methods of establishing and monitoring acceptable standards of clinical practice. National and international organizations and societies in many countries are concerned with supporting research and education in this field and these bodies include the Anesthesia Patient Safety Foundation in the United States, The International Committee on Prevention of Anesthesia Mortality and Morbidity, and the Australian Patient Safety Foundation.

# Audit of clinical anaesthesia

There are several components to the delivery of anaesthesia and these can be analysed in terms of structure, process and outcome (Donabedian, 1988).

## Structural assessment

This encompasses those elements necessary for delivery of anaesthesia to be possible and includes the equipment, facilities, personnel and system of administration.

### Equipment

Both international and British standards cover aspects of anaesthetic machine design, evaluation and approval (Richardson, 1988; Schneider, 1988; Schwanbom, 1988). Although modern anaesthetic machine design continues to improve (Thompson, 1987), many potentially serious problems that occur during an anaesthetic are related to equipment. Older machines are able to deliver a hypoxic mixture, something that is never needed during an anaesthetic, and the inadequacy of breathing systems connections is reflected in the large number of reported disconnection incidents. Other equipment for anaesthetic care, resuscitation and surgery must be of the appropriate design and quality. All equipment must be correctly serviced and maintained and obsolete or worn out apparatus replaced.

### Personnel

Staff must be available in sufficient numbers on all occasions, and be properly trained and qualified to perform their tasks. This includes medical, nursing and ancillary staff. Professional and trade bodies set standards with respect to training, supervision and responsibilities, and there should be systems to ensure review of training and quality of work within each department.

Most preventable anaesthetic-related major morbidity and mortality is caused by human error. The behaviour involved in making errors is essentially normal (Chappelow, 1988) and indeed can result from the automation of simple actions and mental processes that arise from training and experience. Factors including fatigue, anxiety and boredom may degrade performance and make mistakes more likely. Equipment design and environmental conditions, such as noise levels and ambient light and temperature, can alter the likelihood of accidents occurring.

*Anaesthetists*

The College of Anaesthetists is the academic body with responsibility in the United Kingdom for maintaining standards of anaesthetic practice. The College achieves this through the setting of examinations, supervision of appointments, inspection of posts and educational activities. It is a source of advice to many bodies, including central government. Responsibility for education is assumed by advisers at regional level and tutors at district level. The Quality of Practice Committee of the College of Anaesthetists recommends that all anaesthetic trainees keep a log book of their anaesthetic activities as an aid towards assessing adequacy of training. All British anaesthetists are required to pass a three part specialist examination before being allowed to proceed to 'Higher Training'. The Higher Professional Training (HPT) is overseen by the Joint Committee for Higher Training of Anaesthetists and consists of representatives of the College of Anaesthetists, The Scottish Standing Committee of the College, the Faculty of Anaesthetists of the Royal College of Surgeons of Ireland, the Association of Anaesthetists of Great Britain and Ireland, and the Association of University Professors of Anaesthesia. The Committee will ensure that the trainee completes the required period of Higher Training in approved posts and is then able to recommend to the College of Anaesthetists that a Certificate of Accreditation be granted. This Certificate is recognition of the holder's eligibility for consultant responsibility, although it does not carry any guarantee of appointment to that grade. Other professional bodies, notably the Association of Anaesthetists in the United Kingdom, may represent views of anaesthetists and participate in the formation of opinions and policy as well as contributing to education and the formulation of practice standards.

In the United Kingdom, once an anaesthetist is appointed to a consultant post, there is at present no formal assessment or compulsory continuing education. In other countries renewal of a licence to practise is dependent on evidence of participation in such programmes, as well as the maintenance of clinical skills. It would seem reasonable to do the same in the United Kingdom.

Administering an anaesthetic has sometimes been compared to flying an aircraft – 95% boredom and 5% sheer terror. The qualities needed to be an airline pilot are similar in many ways to those of an anaesthetist – judgement, team work, practical skills, the ability to carry out several activities at once and the ability to prioritize competing demands when under pressure. The selection and training of pilots compares interestingly with that of anaesthetists (Butler, 1988). The pilot in training has to undergo tests of practical skills and will participate in formal group activity tasks to assess qualities of judgement and leadership. The professional assessors themselves receive training for the task of assessment to ensure standardization and fairness. Training is structured and progressive from ground school up through simulators to actual flying. The qualified pilot is then subject throughout his career to competency checks and compulsory refresher courses, especially when employed on new aircraft or routes. By comparison, the selection of anaesthetists in the United Kingdom is haphazard and amateur, training is unstructured and without a clear goal, and ongoing assessment patchy or nonexistent. Nor is there compulsory training before employing new apparatus or techniques.

This situation should be viewed along with evidence that a significant proportion of medical graduates have serious psychological disabilities which they carry into medical practice. It appears that certain personalities select given specialties and, compared to other hospital doctors, relatively few anaesthetists appear to be neurotic and anxious individuals; they are also tough minded, practical and intelligent. More importantly, if training and selection within anaesthesia is to improve, there is evidence that the use of psychological testing and trained interviewers can go a long way towards identifying suitable candidates for a career in anaesthesia (Vickers and Reeves, 1990).

*Facilities*

Recommendations on appropriate facilities are made by the Department of Health in the United Kingdom, professional organizations and other bodies. These include details such as operating theatre layout, minimum anaesthetic gas pollution levels and requirements for recovery rooms and high dependency units. Some of these recommendations are ideal goals towards which progress should be made. Organizational standards to define a good acute hospital have been developed (King's Fund Centre for Heath Service Development, 1989) but as yet there is no national scheme to ensure that hospitals reach a given standard in any particular area.

**Process assessment**

This is an examination of the way in which care is provided. To carry out the assessment performance criteria are chosen and indicators selected, such as treatments administered, tests ordered or steps taken to manage specific types of patient or situations, that will show how well practice conforms to the criteria. In this way it should be possible to identify departmental procedures and protocols that could be improved, or individuals whose practice should be changed or can serve as an example to others. For example it may be agreed that monitoring for all patients should be in accordance with the published standards of the Association of Anaesthetists, that all obstetric patients receiving a general anaesthetic are intubated or that a defined anaesthetic machine check should be performed before every anaesthetic session. It may be decided that no more than a given percentage of day care patients having general anaesthesia should be admitted to hospital overnight, that no patient should normally have to stay longer than 2 hours in the postoperative recovery area or that a patient's systolic blood pressure should not inadvertently fall below a systolic of 90 mmHg. In the same way, a statement may be formulated on the number of hours of continuous work or minimum requirements for sleep or rest between cases for anaesthetists. Having laid down the criteria, data are gathered to see how well clinical practice conforms to the agreed or accepted criteria. This can be done in several ways, including a review of anaesthetic charts, or retrospective and prospective surveys.

Assessment of certain aspects of the process of anaesthesia will probably be undertaken on a continuing basis but selected aspects of practice may be examined for a limited period. Problems that occur within a particular group of patients may be picked for scrutiny (Morgan et al., 1983), or aspects of workload and organization analysed (Taylor et al., 1969; Laurenson and Gibbs, 1984). An important part of the process is to feed the information gathered back to the clinicians so that practice can be improved where necessary. The process of assessment is itself beneficial in that it requires a critical analysis of anaesthetic practice to identify the required performance criteria, increases awareness of the selected topics among the staff, and is educational by stimulating discussion and by generating relevant information on work practices. Care must be taken to ensure that clinicians do not feel threatened by the process and it should be carried out in a sensitive and non-accusatory manner in the spirit of wishing first and foremost to increase the quality of care provided to patients.

One method of assessing processes is to undertake peer review of the records of anaesthetics given by others in the department. Records may be selected on a random basis or identified by adverse outcome or other anaesthetic-related factors. A technique developed in Las Vegas (Vitez, 1989) is to review all records where performance did not reach previously agreed standards. One such standard is that ASA I patients should not suffer organ damage or death. When a patient suffers this complication the anaesthetic record is encoded to remove all information that might identify the patient and anaesthetist and it is then reviewed by a Quality Assessment Committee. Any errors that occurred are identified and graded by severity of the sequelae. The errors are then subdivided into categories such as airway, circulatory, regional etc., and a judgement is made as to whether the problem was unavoidable, a mechanical error, or related to human factors. Human errors are further analysed and an attempt is made to explain the origin of the error. The analysis can then be discussed with the anaesthetist responsible and the frequency with which problems arise can identify shortcomings in practice, both by an individual but also within a group. Improvements may then be possible through education, training, supervision, the use of protocols or the provision of equipment and facilities (Gaba, Maxwell and Deanda, 1987). Human error is the cause of perhaps 80% of the incidents and it is likely that many of these incidents arise because of temporary, atypical lapses in the vigilance of otherwise competent anaesthetists. A review of human factors in accidents seen from an aviation viewpoint (Allnutt, 1987) provides a fascinating insight into the process. We all make errors, and recognizing this is an important step towards preventing disaster.

## Outcome assessment

Surveys and reports of anaesthetic risk identify the frequency of certain outcomes and may help identify factors that contribute to morbidity and mortality (Derrington and Smith, 1987; Holland, 1987; Morgan, 1987). Many published articles in anaesthetic journals are a form of audit of this sort. For example, the comparative effect of premedicants may be studied, or recovery from different anaesthetic techniques compared (Forrest *et al.*, 1990). Assessment of outcome also encompasses critical incident analysis, which examines events that if not detected would have led to an adverse outcome.

## Case reports

Some events are so rare or so obvious that case reports remain the best method of identifying an area of anaesthetic concern. The dangers of using bupivacaine for intravenous regional anaesthesia (IVRA, Biers block) were suggested by several case reports of deaths with this technique (Heath, 1982). One of the factors common to all the cases was the use of bupivacaine, and this stimulated much subsequent research demonstrating the cardiotoxicity of this agent and the potential hazards of IVRA. On the basis of this information, bupivacaine was withdrawn for use with this technique and recommendations published on the method of performing this block. A more recent example examines the risk of sedation given to patients receiving a spinal anaesthetic (Caplan *et al.*, 1988). A warning is given of a potential danger with this combination and a hypothesis is put forward to explain this increased risk.

## Critical incident analysis

Critical incident analysis has been developed for use in anaesthesia by Cooper and his colleagues (Cooper *et al.*, 1978). A critical incident is defined as an occurrence that could have led, if not discovered in time, or did lead, to an undesirable patient outcome ranging from increased duration of hospital stay, to death or permanent disability. In anaesthetic practice the incident should occur when the patient is under anaesthetic care, and either involve an error by the anaesthetic team, or a failure of anaesthetic equipment. Examples include breathing circuit disconnections, administration of the wrong drug and accidental extubation. The number and type of critical incidents is collected by interview, questionnaire or with a prospective survey (Currie, Pybus and Torda, 1988). Up to 50% of patients in theatres and more than 30% of patients in recovery have been reported to be subject to a mishap with a potentially serious outcome. Incidents can be classified and factors contributing to the incidents identified. Although many factors emerge, failure to perform a machine check, lack of experience, supervision and familiarity with equipment, haste and fatigue seem to be important. Having identified the reasons for the incidents, action can be taken to prevent further occurrence, indeed a list of strategies to prevent or detect critical incidents has been suggested (Table 8.1) (Cooper, Newbower and Kitz, 1984). In one study the occurrence of critical incidents was reduced from 1 : 160 anaesthetics to 1 : 353 by means of improved feedback, the replacement of old anaesthetic machines and the introduction of a formal anaesthesia apparatus checklist (Kumar *et al.*, 1988). Other valuable information can be gained such as the identification of 'pivotal factors' that warn of a critical incident. An example, from cases reviewed before the general use of oximetry and capnography, is that a change in pulse or blood pressure secondary to hypoxia was the commonest warning of a breathing circuit disconnection. Data such as this strongly support the use of ventilator alarms, oximetry and capnography.

Table 8.1    Strategies to prevent or detect critical incidents

1.  Additional training
2.  Organizational improvements
3.  Improved supervision/second opinion
4.  Equipment/additional monitoring
5.  Equipment or apparatus inspection
    More complete preoperative assessment
    Improved communication
6.  Specific protocols
    Improved personnel selection

Listed in order of importance. After Cooper, Newbower and Kitz (1984).

## Review of morbidity and mortality

Some of the specific risk factors associated with anaesthesia have been discussed earlier (Chapter 2). Important factors include preoperative health (e.g. ASA physical status), major pre-existing cardiovascular, respiratory, renal, hepatic, vascular, metabolic or endocrine disease, advanced age, obesity, major surgery and emergency procedures. Major epidemiological studies in the United Kingdom include the triennial Confidential Enquiry into Maternal Deaths, the study of Lunn and Mushin (1982) and the Confidential Enquiry into Perioperative Deaths (CEPOD) (Buck, Devlin and Lunn, 1987). Approximately one death per 10 000 operations is attributable solely to anaesthesia, and anaesthesia also contributes to another three or four deaths per 10 000. Most recent papers suggest that this mortality rate may be falling (Buck, Devlin and Lunn, 1987; Holland, 1987). It is thought that perhaps 80% or more of the deaths solely due to anaesthesia may be preventable. The factors that contribute to anaesthetic mortality remain depressingly constant (Table 8.2). The recommendations based on these studies reach similar conclusions (Table 8.3). The CEPOD report demonstrated that much postoperative mortality was contributed to by surgical factors. These factors included inadequate preoperative assessment, the operations being performed by an inappropriate surgeon, or the performance of an unnecessary operation. Several important recommendations ensue from this report, including the need for quality assurance or audit.

**Table 8.2   Factors contributing to mortality**

*Before operation*
Inadequate assessment
Uncorrected hypovolaemia

*During the operation*
Lack of prophylaxis against DVT
Aspiration
Inadequate monitoring
Problems with intubation
Inexperience/lack of supervision
Hypoxic gas mixture
Errors in the management of regional techniques

*Postoperative*
Inadequate patient supervision
Ventilatory failure – opioids/relaxants

**Table 8.3   Recommendations to decrease mortality**

Full preoperative assessment
Adequate resuscitation preoperatively
Making a complete and readable anaesthetic record
Better patient monitoring
Good postoperative recovery rooms and staff

Similar surveys have quantified the incidence of anaesthetic related morbidity, both major and minor (Cohen *et al.*, 1986; Pedersen and Johansen, 1989). Major morbidity, not infrequently, has the same causes and therefore the same solutions as mortality. Major morbidity attributable to anaesthesia has been reported with an incidence of 1 : 170 anaesthetics (Pedersen and Johansen, 1989). The commonest problem was cardiovascular collapse, often at induction and especially with the use of suxamethonium. Regional techniques were associated with several cases of cardiovascular collapse as well as the problem of severe postoperative headache. Awareness is extremely distressing for the patient and accounted for nearly 20% of the cases. Peripheral nerve injury, usually caused by malpositioning, should be a preventable cause of major morbidity. Dental trauma is often preventable and is the commonest reason in the United Kingdom and the United States for litigation against the anaesthetist (Clokie, Metcalf and Holland, 1989). Minor morbidity does not result in permanent sequelae but is none the less often very distressing for the patient, and can prolong the hospital stay. The commonest problems are sore throat, headache and nausea and vomiting (Cohen *et al.*, 1986). A high incidence of muscle pains follows the use of suxamethonium. Many of these minor sequelae can be prevented or ameliorated with care and forethought, and by using appropriate techniques.

# Standards of practice

## *Protocols and standards*

Many bodies exert an influence on professional standards in the United Kingdom (Adams, 1983). They include the General Medical Council, the Universities, the Royal Colleges, their Faculties and, in respect of anaesthesia, the College of Anaesthetists. Other professional bodies include the Association of Anaesthetists of Great Britain and Ireland, and the regional and local societies of anaesthesia. Finally all districts in the National Health Service have a departmental organization, and many regions have an anaesthetics advisory committee.

The use of 'protocols' for treatment of specific conditions is widely accepted. These include recommendations for bacterial prophylaxis, preoperative X-ray screening and suggestions for managing malignant hyperthermia or a failed intubation. Norms and standards of clinical care are being published to cover a much wider range of clinical medicine. Several areas of anaesthetic practice in the United States and also in the United Kingdom are now governed by such standards. These include recommendations for minimal standards of patient monitoring (Chapter 5) and procedures for anaesthetic machine checks (Chapter 4). Standards to cover all aspects of an anaesthetic service would encompass the aims and objectives of the service, the scope of the service, organization and staffing, education, training and staff development, equipment, supplies and facilities, operational policies, accreditation, quality assurance, audit and performance. Although comprehensive standards do not exist, it is possible that they may be formulated in the future (Baldock, 1990).

The Royal College of Surgeons has issued *Guidelines to Clinical Audit in Surgical Practice* (Royal College of Surgeons, 1989), which describes the way in which surgical audit should be performed. The process should include regular meetings, with a written record of attendance and discussion. Meetings should be held during normal working hours and about $1\frac{1}{2}$ hours per week should be set aside for them. The College has also published recommendations for making medical records and notes (Royal College of Surgeons, 1990). These involve anaesthetists, as the records should contain details relating to any anaesthetic given, including preoperative anaesthetic assessment, anaesthetic drugs and doses, monitoring data, fluid administration and postoperative instructions. Participation in audit and accurate clinical records will be necessary for surgical accreditation. Similar recommendations are likely to apply to anaesthetists in the future.

Standards fulfil several functions. They stand as a mark of minimal acceptable practice and thus educate the physician, administrators, lawyers and public. They provide a useful yardstick for comparison with current usage in a hospital and, if necessary, with which to confront managers who do not provide recommended equipment or facilities, and they may also be used to compel colleagues to accept recognized practices. Standards are designed to be widely accepted and achievable and this means that they generally represent the minimum required and, in the pursuit of excellence, standards will be regularly exceeded. If practice falls short of published standards then it becomes difficult to justify, especially in a court of law. In the United States adhering to monitoring standards is rewarded by some insurance companies with a cut in premiums (Zeitlin, 1989), and in order to ensure compliance insurers may impose conditions on clinical practice. For anaesthetists to qualify for a premium discount one company asks that a written promise is made that they will comply with the American Society of Anesthesiologists Standards for Basic Intraoperative Monitoring, use a pulse oximeter on every patient and a capnograph wherever applicable. They must also agree to random audit of compliance by the insurance company.

The concept of reaching an adequate standard of anaesthetic care is more nebulous but has been widely used in outcome studies. This involves physician review of the anaesthetic records and a judgement as to whether the conduct of the anaesthetic contributed to the adverse outcome. In one study reviewing closed malpractice claims (Cheney *et al.*, 1989) care was judged to be inappropriate if 'shortcuts' were taken, if the patient was not appropriately or continuously monitored, if serious errors in judgement were made that affected the patient adversely, or if there was poor choice and/or conduct of the anaesthetic. The validity of this approach is supported by the finding that payments were made in more than 80% of claims where substandard anaesthetic care was judged to have been delivered. However it is sobering to realize that even when the care was felt to be appropriate, payment was made in some 40% of the cases.

Comparing outcome between institutions will indicate if there are gross disparities in standards of treatment. Steps must be taken to standardize factors such as different hospital populations and illness severity. This approach is now widely adopted in the intensive care and trauma literature, with scoring systems such as APACHE II (Knaus et al., 1985) used to standardize severity of illness or injury. If outcomes for the same procedure vary widely between hospitals or even between physicians in the same hospital then further investigation is indicated. For example among 84 surgeons operating for large bowel cancer there was a sixfold variation in the rate of anastomotic breakdown (Fielding et al., 1980) and major morbidity and mortality for carotid endarterectomy in two separate papers was nearly ten times greater in one institution compared to the other (Easton and Sherman, 1977; Sundt et al., 1981). Other examples can also be found (Mortensen, 1989). On a more mundane level, patients under the care of one surgeon may spend twice as long in hospital for the same operation as those being managed by another consultant. In all the examples quoted, it is relevant to find out why the differences exist.

## The effect of standards and audit on outcome

The introduction of minimum standards has undoubtedly influenced clinical practice, although other pressures such as fear of litigation are presumably also important (Cohen, Wade and Woodward, 1990). It is likely that there was a decline in anaesthetic-related mortality over the years before the introduction of formal minimum monitoring standards (Zeitlin, 1989), and this may be due to factors such as better training, education, equipment and assistance for the anaesthetist.

It is impossible to prove conclusively that the new standards have further decreased mortality (Orkin, 1989), but some evidence suggests that this is so. Out of more than one million ASA I and II patients who underwent anaesthesia at one of the Harvard hospitals between 1976 and mid 1988, 11 suffered a major intraoperative accident solely attributable to the conduct of the anaesthetic. It was judged that the seven cases of unrecognized hypoventilation and the single case where oxygen was accidentally discontinued should have been prevented by early warnings that would have been given by the Harvard minimal monitoring standards (Eichhorn, 1989). An associated problem was inadequate supervision of junior and subordinate anaesthetists. From shortly after introduction of the standards in 1985 up to mid 1988, 319 000 anaesthetics were administered without a major preventable intraoperative injury. As another illustration there were 27 major claims concerning hypoxia against one insurance group in the 18 months up to December 1986 but no claims in this category in 1988 when almost all anaesthetists used pulse oximetry and capnography (Pierce, 1989). The introduction of pulse oximetry into operating theatres was probably responsible for significantly decreasing the incidence of so-called 'recovery room impact events', which are unanticipated, undesirable effects under anaesthesia requiring intervention and with relevance to recovery room care (Cooper et al., 1987). The availability of pulse oximetry decreases the number of hypoxic episodes experienced by children undergoing anaesthesia (Coté et al., 1988) and the capnograph has also been shown to be useful in detecting problems relating to ventilation in the paediatric population. Over the past few years, since the adoption of minimal standards, the cost of malpractice claims against anaesthetists in the United States has decreased by some 66% to such an extent that insurance premiums at the nine Harvard Hospitals have been cut by nearly 40%.

The importance of audit is not so much in gathering data on patient outcome, but in the process of feeding back the information when analysed, thereby altering practice where necessary and hopefully improving patient care. It cannot be assumed that information alone will improve practice (Cooper et al., 1987), although it is likely that increased awareness of high risk events will raise the level of vigilance. It is necessary to continue with the audit process to assess the impact of any changes that are made.

Much of the preventable anaesthetic-related mortality is secondary to human error. No amount of monitoring is a substitute for an intelligent, motivated, alert doctor who has been properly trained, is adequately supervised, provided with the right equipment and support, and is not performing beyond his capability. Standards covering work practices are common in other occupations. The maximum number of hours that doctors work is already limited by law in some countries or states (Cooper, 1989). Designated rest periods, minimum acceptable experience, and changes in training and supervision may be recommended for anaesthetists in the future.

# References

Adams, A. K. (1983) Quality assurance in anaesthesia. *Anaesthesia*, **38**, 311–313

Allnutt, M. F. (1987) Human factors in accidents. *British Journal of Anaesthesia*, **59**, 856–864

Baldock, G. J. (1990) Quality assurance, standards and accreditation. *Anaesthesia*, **45**, 617–618

Brown, E. M. (1984) Quality assurance in anesthesiology – the problem-orientated audit. *Anesthesiology*, **63**, 611–615

Buck, N., Devlin, H. B. and Lunn, J. N. (1987) Report of the Confidential Enquiry into Perioperative Deaths (CEPOD). Nuffield Provincial Hospitals Trust/King's Fund, London

Butler, A. J. J. (1988) Safety aspects of personnel selection and training of pilots. In: *Baillière's Clinical Anaesthesiology* (eds. O. P. Dinnick and P. W. Thompson), vol. 2, no. 2, June, Baillière Tindall, London, ch. 2

Caplan, R. A., Posner, K., Ward, R. J. and Cheney, F. W. (1988) Unexpected cardiac arrest during spinal anesthesia: a closed claims analysis of predisposing factors. *Anesthesiology*, **68**, 5–11

Chappelow, J. (1988) The psychology of safety. In: *Baillière's Clinical Anaesthesiology* (eds. O. P. Dinnick and P. W. Thompson), vol. 2, no. 2, June, Baillière Tindall, London, ch. 3

Cheney, F. W., Posner, K. Caplan, R. A. and Ward, R. J. (1989) Standards of care and anesthesia liability. *Journal of the American Medical Association*, **261**, 1599–1603

Clokie, C., Metcalf, I. and Holland, A. (1989) Dental trauma in anaesthesia. *Canadian Journal of Anaesthesia*, **36**, 675–680

Cohen, M. H., Duncan, P. G., Pope, W. D. B. and Wolkenstein, C. (1986) A survey of 112 000 anaesthetics at one teaching hospital. *Canadian Anaesthetists Society Journal*, **33**, 22–31

Cohen, M. M., Wade, J. and Woodward, C. (1990) Medical-legal concerns among Canadian anaesthetists. *Canadian Journal of Anaesthesia*, **37**, 102–111

Cooper, J. B. (1989) Report of a meeting of the International Committee for Prevention of Anesthesia Mortaility and Morbidity. *Anaesthesia*, **44**, 441–443

Cooper, J. B., Cullen, D. J., Nemeskal, R., Hoaglin, D. C., Gervitz, C. C., Csete, M. and Venable, C. (1987) Effects of information feedback and pulse oximetry on the incidence of anesthesia complications. *Anesthesiology*, **67**, 684–694

Cooper, J. B., Newbower, R. S. and Kitz, R. J. (1984) An analysis of major errors and equipment failures in anesthesia management: considerations for prevention and detection. *Anesthesiology*, **60**, 34–42

Cooper, J. B., Newbower, R. S., Long, C. D. and McPeek, B. J. (1978) Preventable anesthesia mishaps – a study in human factors. *Anesthesiology*, **49**, 399–406

Coté, C. J., Goldstein, E. A., Cote, M. A., Hoaglin, D. C. and Ryan, J. F. (1988) A single-blind study of pulse oximetry in children. *Anesthesiology*, **68**, 184–188

Currie, M., Pybus, D. A. and Torda, T. A. (1988) A prospective survey of anaesthetic critical events: a report of a pilot study of 88 cases. *Anaesthesia and Intensive Care*, **16**, 1103–1106

Derrington, M. C. and Smith, G. (1987) A review of studies of anaesthetic risk, morbidity and mortality. *British Journal of Anaesthesia*, **59**, 815–833

Donabedian, A. (1988) The quality of care. How can it be assessed? *Journal of the American Medical Association*, **260**, 1743–1748

Easton, J. D. and Sherman, D. G. (1977) Stroke and mortality rate in carotid endarterectomy: 228 consecutive operations. *Stroke*, **8**, 565–568

Eichhorn, J. H. (1989) Prevention of intraoperative anesthesia accidents and related severe injury through safety monitoring. *Anesthesiology*, **70**, 572–577

Fielding, L. P., Stewart-Brown, S., Blesovsky, L. and Kearney, G. (1980) Anastomotic integrity after operations for large bowel cancer: a multicentre study. *British Medical Journal*, **281**, 411–414

Forrest, J. B., Cahalan, M. K., Rehder, K., Goldsman, C. H., Levy, W. J., Strunin, L., Bota, W., Boucek, C. D., Cucchiara, R. F., Dhamee, S., Domino, K. B., Dudman, A. J. U., Hamilton, W. K., Kampine, J., Kotrly, K. J., Maltby, J. R., Mazlookdoost, M., Mackenzie, R. A., Melnick, B. M., Motoyama, E., Muir, J. J. and Munshi, C. (1990) Multicenter study of general anesthesia II. Results. *Anesthesiology*, **72**, 262–268

Gaba, D. M., Maxwell, M. and Deanda, A. (1987) Anesthetic mishaps: breaking the chain of accident evolution. *Anesthesiology*, **66**, 670–676

Heath, M. L. (1982) Deaths after intravenous regional anaesthesia. *British Medical Journal*, **2**, 913–914

Holland, R. (1987) Anaesthetic mortality in New South Wales. *British Journal of Anaesthesia*, **59**, 834–841

King's Fund Centre for Health Service Development (1989) *Guidelines for Standards in Acute Hospitals*. Quality Assurance Programme, London

Knaus, W. A., Draper, E. A., Wagner, D. P. and Zimmerman, J. E. (1985) APACHE II: severity of disease classification system. *Critical Care Medicine*, **13**, 818–829

Kumar, V., Barcellos, W. A., Mehta, M. P. and Carter, J. G. (1988) An analysis of critical incidents in a teaching department for quality assurance. A survey of mishaps during anaesthesia. *Anaesthesia*, **43**, 879–883

Laurenson, V. G. and Gibbs, J. M. (1984) A computer-based audit of anaesthetic registrar training. *Anaesthesia and Intensive Care*, **12**, 152–154

Lunn, J. N. and Mushin, W. W. (1982) Mortality associated with anaesthesia. Nuffield Provincial Hospitals Trust, London

Morgan, B. M., Abulakh, J. M., Barker, J. P., Goroszeniuk, T. and Trojanowski, A. (1983) Anaesthesia for caesarean section. A medical audit of junior anaesthetic staff practice. *British Journal of Anaesthesia*, **55**, 885–889

Morgan, M. (1987) Anaesthetic contribution to maternal mortality. *British Journal of Anaesthesia*, **59**, 842–855

Mortensen, N. (1989) Wide variations in surgical mortality. Standard definition needed for postoperative mortality. *British Medical Journal*, **298**, 344–345

Orkin, F. K. (1989) Practice standards: the Midas touch or the Emperor's new clothes? *Anesthesiology*, **70**, 567–571

Pedersen, T. and Johansen, S. H. (1989) Serious morbidity attributable to anaesthesia. Considerations for prevention. *Anaesthesia*, **44**, 504–508

Pierce, E. C., Jr. (1989) Anesthesia: standards of care and liability. *Journal of the American Medical Association*, **262**, 773

Report of the Standard Medical Advisory Committee (1990) The Quality of Medical Care. HMSO, London

Richardson, N. H. (1988) Medical equipment regulation and the role of the test house. In: *Baillière's Clinical Anaesthesiology* (eds. O. P. Dinnick and P. W. Thompson), vol. 2, no. 2, June, Baillière Tindall, London, ch. 9

Royal College of Surgeons of England (1989) *Guidelines to Clinical Audit in Surgical Practice.* RCS, London

Royal College of Surgeons of England (1990) *Guidelines for Clinicians on Medical Records and Notes.* RCS, London

Schneider, A. J. L. (1988) Regulation of anaesthesia devices in the United States. In: *Baillière's Clinical Anaesthesiology* (eds. O. P. Dinnick and P. W. Thompson), vol. 2, no. 2, June, Baillière Tindall, London, ch. 8

Schwanbom, E. (1988) Does safe design guarantee safety? In: *Baillière's Clinical Anaesthesiology* (eds. O. P. Dinnick and P. W. Thompson), vol. 2, no. 2, June, Baillière Tindall, London, ch. 7

Shaw, C. D. (1980) Aspects of audit. Looking forward to audit. *British Medical Journal*, **1**, 1509–1511

Sundt, T. M., Sharbrough, F. W., Piepgras, D. G., Kearns, T. P., Messick, J. M., Jr. and O'Fallon, W. M. (1981) Correlation of cerebral blood flow and electroencephalographic changes during carotid endarterectomy. *Mayo Clinic Proceedings*, **56**, 533–543

Taylor, T. H., Jennings, A. M. C., Nightingale, D. A., Barker, B., Leivers, D., Styles, M. and Magner, J. (1969) Study of anaesthetic emergency work II: the work of the three hospitals. *British Journal of Anaesthesia*, **41**, 76–83

Thompson, P. W. (1987) Safer design of anaesthetic equipment. *British Journal of Anaesthesia*, **59**, 913–921

Vickers, M. D. and Reeves, P. E. (1990) Selection methods in medicine: a case for replacement surgery? *Journal of the Royal Society of Medicine*, **83**, 541–543

Vitez, T. S. (1989) Effective quality assessment system developed. *American Society of Anesthesiologists Newsletter*, **53**, 8–10

Working for Patients (1989) Working Paper no. 6, Cmnd 555, HMSO, London

Zeitlin, G. L. Possible decrease in mortality associated with anaesthesia. A comparison of two time periods in Massachusetts, USA. *Anaesthesia*, **44**, 432–433

# 9

# Standards of care: the good, the bad and the acceptable

Simon Taylor

## Introduction

This chapter examines the way in which the law courts approach medical negligence cases. A contrast is drawn between the standards of care to which the profession aspires and the standards which must be attained to avoid a finding of negligence. The limitations which should be put upon the use of this book in a medicolegal context are examined.

## The need for expert evidence

Disputes in court cases are decided on the evidence presented to the court. The usual rule is that the evidence should be of facts, not opinions. This rule works well in many cases in which there is an allegation of negligence. In, for example, a case involving a road accident the judge needs to know the speeds, directions of travel and positions of the vehicles, the road conditions and so on. With that factual evidence he can decide who was to blame. The opinion of a witness that X was to blame is not generally admitted in evidence, although the exclusion of such evidence, particularly where the witness was not involved in the accident and is himself an experienced driver, can be hard to justify.

However, the subject matter of the case may be so far removed from the judge's experience that to expect him to try the case having heard only factual evidence would be absurd. Medical negligence cases fall into this category, and may turn on expert evidence.

---

Throughout this chapter the masculine pronoun has been used for convenience only. No sexual stereotyping is implied.

In these cases the facts are established by evidence from the patient, and from friends or relatives, doctors, nurses and other staff present at the material times, and by reference to medical records, X-rays and other documents. Based on this evidence the judge makes findings of fact (e.g. 'The explanation given to the patient was that . . .' or 'The dose of morphine given was . . .'). The expert evidence, usually given by distinguished – or at least experienced – doctors practising in the appropriate field, can bear on the facts. Thus where there are conflicting versions of the facts, an expert may pronounce on which version he thinks is more likely to be correct. Or, the expert may be asked to interpret accepted facts such as the results of a blood test. However, the expert's primary role is to state whether *in his opinion* a particular act or omission was negligent. That opinion will in most cases be founded on the expert's own experience fortified by reference to medical literature and standard textbooks.

## Impugning expert evidence

Experts giving evidence on any of these aspects of a case may disagree amongst themselves. Where such disagreement relates to matters peculiarly within their expertise (i.e. where the expert is stating an opinion rather than hypothesizing as to the existence of a fact) the judge is put in an awkward position. He cannot become an expert himself and say that the evidence of one expert is, in the judge's opinion, clearly right, while the evidence of the other is wrong. This difficulty is to some extent recognized by the *Bolam* test (*Bolam* v. *Friern Hospital Management Committee* [1957] 2 All ER 118) which states that a doctor is not negligent if he acts in accordance with a practice accepted as proper a responsible body of men skilled in the particular field in question, merely because there is a body of opinion that takes a contrary view. It may, in some circumstances, be possible to define the best practice. Equally there may be circumstances in which the medical care given would be universally condemned as unacceptable. In between these extremes is practice which is considered acceptable: this category may include treatment in a given situation which one doctor will say is wrong but which another will endorse as correct. The *Bolam* test comes into its own in relation to this middle category: if the patient's experts say that a doctor was negligent, but the doctor's experts say that he was not, then in general a judge will be constrained to find in favour of the doctor. It is usually necessary, therefore, if a medical negligence case is contested, for the patient's lawyers, with the assistance of their experts, to attack the foundation of the expert opinions given in support of the doctor, by, for example, disputing that the 'expert's' field of expertise covers the issues in the case, or by pointing out flaws in his reasoning. As a matter of theory this attack on the other side's experts could perhaps be avoided by the doctor's lawyers – who merely have to show that there is a responsible body of medical opinion which supports their client's actions – but in practice the same assault on the expertise of the 'expert' or on the cogency of his opinion is likely to be made by both sides.

The undermining of an expert opinion is sometimes achieved by a logical dissection of what has been said by the expert. Thus where an expert has said that fact A implies fact B, but has forgotten to take into account fact C (which is relevant) his conclusion may be invalid. Another approach to the problem of attacking a contrary expert opinion is to show that it does not take into account, or differs from, the views expressed in the relevant literature. It is in this context, and others, that a book such as this, entitled *Standards of Care in Anaesthesia*, is both useful and open to misuse. Of course, the primary purpose of this present book is not medico-legal: it is written for the education – in a broad sense – of doctors. It does, however, have proper medico-legal uses: it may indicate lines of enquiry both in the preparation of a case and, with experts guiding the lawyers, at trial. What it cannot do – and does not purport to do – is lay down rules as to how an anaesthetist must act.

## The judge's task

In most medical negligence cases a judge will be called upon to decide what constitutes a reasonable standard of care in a particular situation. He has to apply an objective test, so that the performance of all doctors facing a given set of circumstances is likely to be judged by reference to the same (minimum) standard of conduct. The judge, being in medical terms a layman, cannot set that standard (and thereby decide the case) without expert assistance. He may, however, be assailed by different opinions as to what was reasonable conduct in the circumstances from experts each of whom has an impeccable pedigree in terms of qualifications and experience. How tempting it would then be to fall back on written guidelines for the conduct of doctors, and to treat a book entitled 'Standards of Care in . . .' as such guidelines! That would not, of course, be the correct approach, for it would in all probability give insufficient weight to the facts of the particular case. For example, a court should not find negligence in every case in which a cardiac monitor was not used during anaesthesia; but if a judge or other layman were to thumb through this book, the wealth of information on monitoring might drive him to the erroneous conclusion that it is (medically speaking) mandatory. The example illustrates the importance in a medico-legal context of examining the particular facts before reaching a conclusion, and of taking appropriate expert advice on those facts rather than relying on expertise expressed in general terms in a textbook.

# Regulation and medical practice

The injunction against using a reference book as a rule book should not lead to the conclusion that written standards of conduct are irrelevant in negligence cases, for noncompliance with what may be termed codes of practice or with the procedures advocated by a venerated textbook can be highly probative of a failure to reach a reasonable standard of care. In some jurisdictions, though not in England and Wales, the legislature has made rules for the conduct of an anaesthetic, thus enshrining professional standards as law. Parliament has seen fit to take this sort of approach in almost every industrial setting, giving directions not only as to the design of the workplace but also as to the tools to be used and the mode of work. A good example is the Jute (Safety, Health and Welfare) Regulations 1948, which apply to any factory in which jute is spun or woven: in relation to the workplace it is specified that in any workroom the ends of every steam-heated cylinder used in connection with a dressing machine shall be kept effectively covered with insulating material in good repair in such manner as to prevent, so far as is reasonably practicable, the escape of heat therefrom; and in relation to the machinery it is specified that (on carding and teasing machines) the in-running nip between the delivery roller and the pressing ball shall be securely fenced throughout its length; and in relation to the mode of work it is specified that a woman aged 18 years or over may carry (by herself) a maximum weight of material of 65 lb as a reasonably compact or rigid body and 50 lb when it is not a reasonably compact or rigid body (which are the same weights allowed to be carried by a male aged 16 years but under 18).

In a medical context, however, statutory regulation (at least in the United Kingdom) has not gone nearly so far. Analogous provisions relating to the design of operating theatres, and to the design of anaesthetic machines exist. The third aspect of industrial regulation quoted (the regulation of the mode of working), which is meant to protect employees from harm, has no equivalent in the practice of medicine. Regulating employers in order to protect employees is thought to be necessary and practicable, but regulating clinical practice in order to protect patients is not. This *laissez-faire* attitude is unlikely to be immutable. Indeed, if the term 'clinical practice' is given a wide meaning then it can be seen that there is already, or that there is soon likely to be, a good deal of regulation, whether by legislation or by contractual arrangements applicable to all doctors working within the National Health Service.

The regulation referred to goes well beyond simply cutting doctors' hours. Obvious areas in which there is already statutory regulation impinging on clinical practice include the prescribing of drugs and the carrying out of therapeutic abortions. Less obviously, the process by which the professional bodies accredit certain hospitals and posts within them as suitable for training junior doctors, is in a sense, regulation of clinical practice. So too, in a sense, is the government's policy of stipulating (by means of contractual arrangements) the facilities and health checks which a general practitioner must offer to his patients. Professional customs are also, in some ways, regulatory: it is now rare in the United Kingdom, for example, for an anaesthetic to be given without some form of monitoring. But at the heart of clinical practice lies clinical decision-making – the moment when the doctor asks himself 'How do I advise this patient?' or 'What treatment shall I recommend?' or 'What do I do now?' – and it is that process which is not yet regulated in the United Kingdom. It is submitted, moreover, that the moment when a decision has to be made is not truly amenable to regulation, not only because such regulation would be anathema to the medical profession but also because any such regulations would be excessively detailed, hard to devise, difficult to update and impossible to enforce.

A policy of nonregulation is, however, compatible with attempts, sometimes stimulated by government, to maintain and improve professional standards. Properly conducted audit giving rise to recommendations can be highly influential. Thus, for example, the Confidential Enquiry into Perioperative Deaths has, it is to be hoped, been studied in every surgical and anaesthetic department in the country. It, and other forms of audit, should set attainable goals. To expect 'best practice' in every setting is unrealistic, but an audit which defines by consensus what is acceptable practice has some chance of eliminating the unacceptable.

## Conclusion

On the whole, therefore, in the United Kingdom both Parliament and the professional bodies have avoided regulating clinical decision-making, while seeking to maintain standards of practice by the methods discussed. It is these standards of care, set essentially by the profession, which are likely to be presented to a court of law by an expert as the minimum acceptable standards and which are likely to form the basis of the court's decision when deciding whether treatment was negligent or not.

This present book does not seek to pre-empt the court's decision. It is not an attempt merely to define the negligent/non-negligent divide. It describes not simply what is acceptable practice, but what is the *best*. The question may none the less arise, however, of whether a failure to meet the standards set in this book is negligent. That question can only be answered on a case by case basis, by a judge who has determined the facts and heard expert opinions. It would be foolish of lawyers, therefore, to consider using this book or any reference book – however tempting its title – as a quasi-statutory document setting the minimum standards of care.

# Index